Socio-Economic Analysis of Nurses

Socio-Economic Analysis of Nurses

Subhransubala Mohanty

2001

Daya Publishing House
Delhi - 110 035

ISBN 81-7035-243-6

This publication is partly supported by the UGC

Published by : **Daya Publishing House**
1123/74, Deva Ram Park,
Tri Nagar, Delhi - 110 035
Phone : 7199029
Fax : (011) 7198902
e-mail : dayabooks@vsnl.com
website : www.dayabooks.com

Laser Typesetting : **Classic Computer Services**
Delhi - 110 035

Printed at : **Chawla Offset Printers**
Delhi - 110 052

PRINTED IN INDIA

Dedicated to

My

Father

Preface

The study of socio-economic status of nurses is felt as an urgent need to save mankind, who are the part of the Health Care System of the country. Especially in the modern context of industrialisation, the danger to natural environment and its result in human body needs a proper Health Care System. When the environment changes drastically, many human diseases erupt which are detrimental to human existence. In this context, the role of nurses, doctors and all medical agents is very much vital to protect Health Care System of the country as well as the whole world.

This book is a comprehensive treatment of the subject–matter relating to status of medical colleges in Orissa, socio-economic character of nurses and working and living conditions of nurses consisting of six chapters and bibliography. During the preparation of this book the author always remain conscious about the difficulties of nurses and at every step efforts are made to dilute the problems of nurses. Despite the serious efforts, reader may come across the shortcomings of different densities in the book.

The author expresses her thanks to her research guide Dr D.D. Panigrahi, Ex Deputy Director, Directorate of Secondary Education, Orissa and very much indebted to Mrs Sita Mehre, Ex Secretary, Orissa Nursing Employees Association (ONEA); Chief Matron, SCB Medical College, Cuttack; Assistant Matron; MKCG Medical College, Berhampur; Assistant Matron, VSS Medical College, Burla and authorities of the libraries of the Orissa University of Agriculture and Technology (OUAT), Parija Library of Utkal University, Harekrishna Mahatab State Library, Library of Soochana Bhawan, State Museum and seminary library of Post Graduate Department of Economics, Utkal University, Bhubaneswar, Orissa for the permission to utilise.

The author considers her sincere efforts to be amply rewarded if the literature serves the needs of the researchers, sociologists, students and trainees in particular to the best of their advantage.

The author is very much thankful to the publisher, Daya Publishing House for their whole hearted co-operation in the publication of this book. Suggestions for further improvement will be thankfully received and acknowledged.

Subhransubala Mohanty

Contents

List of Tables

List of Figures

Chapter 1
Introductory

1.1 Introduction

"Health for all" by A.D. 2000 and attaining it through primary health care has been the motto of many developing countries in the world today. As many as 166 countries are now busy in evolving strategies to attain this objective by the turn of the country. India is one of the such countries committed to this challenging job and is making all–out efforts to reach this destination. Orissa being one of the poorest and most backward partners in the Indian Union has to make a determined bid to fulfil this laudable national objective. The role of the nursing community assumes importance in the context of such a national endeavour to achieve something which though basic in life, has not been provided for even after four decades of economic planning in the country.

The first step to organise a nursing service by training women for the purpose was taken in Madras in the seventies of the last century. In the following years nurses were introduced in an increasing number of hospitals, the service being established as a general rule with the help of nurses from Western countries. For the large Government hospitals nurses are recruited directly from England, except in some cases nurses belonging to the one or another religious order were invited to organise nursing in a particular hospital. A number of nurses from Europe and America also came to India to work in mission hospitals; their largest contribution to nursing in addition to their example of devotion to duty, has been the training of nurses and midwives which they carried out in the language of the region.

By the beginning of the century, a number of training centres were established mainly in the presidencies of Madras, Bombay and Bengal. Recruitment to nursing was more or less limited to the Anglo–Indian and Christian communities though organisations like the Seva Sadan in Poona encouraged and assisted Hindu women to undergo training in nursing and midwifery. The apprenticeship of training had established. By this process it was confined to mainly hospitals. But the First World War created another field–the Indian Military Nursing Service. Preparation of nursing workers for the public health field was undertaken only in 1918 by the establishment of the Lady Reading Health School for training Health Visitors. During 1920–30 the training of nurses, midwives and health visitors became more standardised and training schools were established in all the provinces of British India and also in many of the Indian states. To improve the standard of nursing and, particularly to prepare nurses for administrative duties in military hospitals, the school of Nursing Administration was established in Delhi by the Government of India in 1945. One of the earliest to be implemented was the Indian Nursing Council Act passed on 31st December, 1947.

After independence, there was considerable development in other fields of health. Social service organisations recognised that training of women for nursing not only provided a needed community service but also, usually, a secure means of livelihood. A completely new feature in 1948 was that instead of an acute shortage of candidates for nursing training there was over the list as because of unexpected stimulus through up–heaval of partition.

1.2 Review of Literature

Few studies have been made on the various aspects of nursing problems in India at the macro level. Authors like Rao (1964), Park (1985) and Bhargav (1987) have analysed the present status of women in society.

Studies have been made at the Government level by the Expert Committees and Commissions like the Bhore Committee (1943), Shetty Committee (1954), Mudaliar Committee (1959) and High Power Committee (1988) on the existing working conditions of nurses and the health care system.

Besides, quite a good number of studies have been made by individual scholars on various issues of nurses. Researchers like Rahudkar (1960), Moore (1978) and Basu (1979) have studied the issues of special stratification and have advocated for a social change.

Studies on social status and its indices, have been made by Reiss (1965) and Bopegamage and Veeraraghban (1967). These studies have dealt with the factors governing the status and images of nurses in the Indian societies in the past and in the changing societies of today.

Similar attempt was also made by Abana (1948), Kind (1968), Berstein (1968), Phillips (1979) and Nagpal (1984) as regards the roles of nurses in different walks of life. They conclude in their studies that reciprocity of society is very much necessary to extract qualitative nursing care from the nursing personnel.

Park (1982) in his studies has discussed issues relating to low socio–economic status of nurses in society and pleads for a fair deal to them in the years to come.

Scholars like Gorwin (1946), Virgina (1961), Levine and Philips (1975), Harner and Lehma (1983), Ranjanna, Shiveran and Vastard (1984), Cruz and Bottorff (1985) have discussed various issues of reorientation of nursing education and advocated for systematic nursing by changing the education pattern and syllabus. Timke *et al.* (1982) and Sweezy *et al.* (1982) have in their studies argued in favour of computerising the nursing education and services.

Report of Geneva Christian medical Commission (1974), United Nation's Report on a Conference (1987), Report of World Health Forum (1987) and Report of World Health Organisation (1988) dealing with the socio–economic problems of nurses have uniformly emphasised on the deleterious effects of heavy work load and poor socio–economic status of nurses and have suggested for a change in the social outlook in this area.

Park (1985) in his study has underlined the health hazards of the nurses in their work place. WHO (1972) has suggested some measures for health protection and restoration at the national level. The Water Act (1984) and Smoke Nuisance Act (1989) are the outcome of it.

1.3 Need of the Study

Basic nursing has its own origin in fundamental and universal human needs regardless of whether a human being is sick or well, the nurse must bear in mind the inherent human needs for food, shelter and clothing, the need for human understanding, underlying all these, is the basic approach to love and to give hope. India is a country of diversified cultures, traditions and habits where nurse has to act as stabilising element to mitigate the suffering which has been accentuated and accelerated.

Dedicated to the service of mankind, nursing is rightly regarded as the noblest of all "callings". The "Sister", as the nurse is affectionately addressed, brings cheers to the sick and suffering and provides invaluable care and service to the patients. She dispels the gloom of suffering with her very presence which rediates hope all around. It can be said that nursing binds the human society with a silken bond of love and affection. It may be taken as a classic example of national integration because the nurse serves all kinds of patients without prejudice of caste, colour, creed, religion or language. Pioneers like Florence Nightingale and Mother Teresa have built up the bridges of international understanding and co–operation with their sense of service and self sacrifice.

Sickness is a companion of man and a sickman needs the nursing care during his period of sickness which is only provided by the nurse in the hospitals. A nurse, therefore, is an indispensable partner of the medical team and a valuable link between the doctors and the patients. Patients, no doubt, get medical advice from the doctors, but they derive a great deal of psychological satisfaction from the services of nurses. Nurse is a productive unit in society the produce being the essential nursing services for the community. Since society makes use of the invaluable services of the nurse is under obligation to provide her in return some facilities commensurate with her service for society. The quality of her services are directly influenced by her working and living conditions. Satisfactory working condition may lead to maximisation of excellent nursing services which, in its turn, can improve the standard of health and welfare of the community.

In the context of national development, participation of nurses in the economic activities is of crucial importance. But the definition and quantification of their work still remains one of the baffling issues in their services. They have also to bear sometimes incalculable and invisible family liabilities mostly not taken into account as is done in case of other working women. The drudgery of domestic work compounded when they reach their work place to shoulder the burden of their duties with its concomitant physical and mental pressure. But the wage they receive is not considered to be commensurate with the mental and physical labour they undergo.

Both the Government and social organisations owe a debt to this noble profession and have an obligation to take up their cause. What follows in this study is an effort to examine thoroughly whether the Government of Orissa is actually providing satisfactory working conditions for the nursing personnel in the State and what the government and society could do to remove the deficiencies so as to bridge the wide gap that exists today between theory and practice of nursing. The government organisation being the largest and the government being a model employer, the responsibility of ensuring better working and living conditions as well as rational income structure naturally devolves upon the government. Lack of social recognition and economic exploitation erode the prestige and status of nurses in our society which in turn gradually deteriorate the quality, competence and morale of the nursing profession in the country today. This calls for a reformation and restructuring of the nursing profession and a change in the environment in which she works. Of course, an unexpectedly high level of income may create a sense of euphoria and unusually low level of income may be a source of embarrassment and a direct cause of their economic hardship. Their efficiency will improve if they are given the status they really deserve in society. This, therefore, needs to be the prime concern of society and the government of the land.

Apart from these surveys, some studies on different aspects of the problems of nursing are in progress at Industrial medical Centre, Lignite Corporation Limited, Neyveli (Personal Communication). These are "Collecting design for nurses in India", "Backache relating to nursing", "Prevalence of Communication", "Contact dermatitis among nurses", "Social problems of nurses in the community"; "Shifts and its effects in nursing profession" and

"Dual roles of nurses as working staff and mother in the family: A cross section study".

It is, thus, observed that the available studies on various aspects of nursing problems have been made almost at the macro level and only a few are available at the micro level.

In Orissa, studies pertaining to the problem of nurses are almost non–existent. No enquiry committee has been formed to study the problem and quantify the degree of exploitation of nurses in the state. Furthermore, no attempt has also so far been made to study the socio–economic problems of nurses. This study has, therefore, been undertaken to throw some light on the various socio –economic problems of nurses in the medical college hospitals of the state and help the state government in formulating appropriate policies to build up an efficient and effective nursing services.

1.4 Objectives and Hypotheses

The objectives of this study are:

1. To assess the social status and dignity accorded to the nursing profession in the present day society and in that context assess and evaluate their economic and working conditions in the medical college hospitals in Orissa.
2. To evaluate the policy measures of the Government of Orissa and suggest measures to uplift the socio–economic status of the nursing community in the state.

The study is based on the following hypotheses:

1. The nurses in the three medical college hospitals in Orissa are enjoying a social status quite befitting to their profession and are working with dignity and that adequate steps have been taken by the government to enhance their socio–economic status in society.
2. Their working conditions are satisfactory and the pay and perks they receive are commensurate with their contribution to the suffering humanity.

1.5 Methodology

The study is mainly persued with primary data and materials collected from the three medical college hospitals by canvassing a detailed questionnaire to the nurses of different categories on the various aspects of their life, living and working conditions, service prospects, economic and social status etc. The stratified census method is followed for the purpose. The data thus collected have been processed scientifically and statistically analysed to draw conclusion on the hypotheses. Collection has been made from the Directorate of Health Services, Orissa, Offices of the Superintendents of the three hospitals and the Secretary Orissa Nursing Employees Association (ONEA). Besides published materials available from various research journals and standard literature have also been extensively used. The views of top level government officials connected with the handling of the administrative problems of the nurses and formulation of policies regarding their conditions of services etc. have been elicited by personal interviews, correspondences and discussions and have been incorporated at appropriate places.

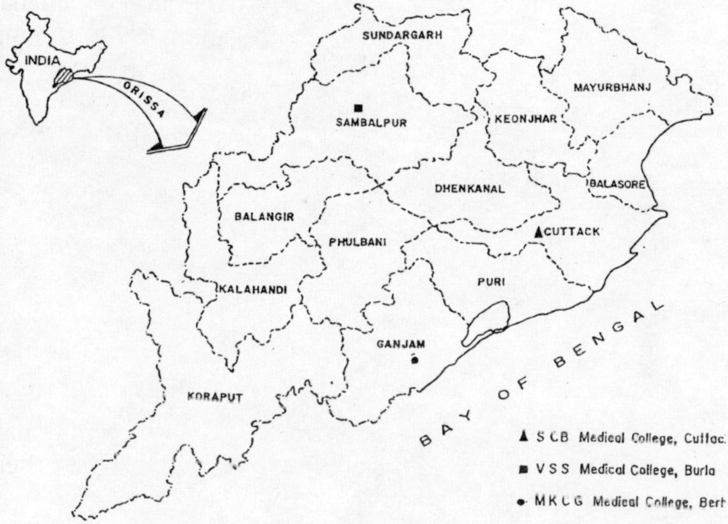

Fig. 1: Map of Orissa showing Study Sites

1.6 Scope of the Study

The scope of the study is confined to the three medical college hospitals of Orissa, *i.e.*, SCB Medical College hospital Cuttack; VSS Medical College hospital, Burla and MKCG Medical College hospital, Berhampur (Fig. 1). It highlights the socio–economic conditions of nurses in these three medical college hospitals. In Orissa, the number of nurses working in the private nursing homes and dispensaries constitute 44.3 per cent of the total nursing population and 21.9 per cent of the total nursing cadre serve only in these three medical college hospitals. Since these are the three premier medical institutions of the state, the working conditions in these institutions may be taken to be representative in character in reflecting the conditions of service of the nursing community of the whole State and a study of their condition would reasonably reflect the general conditions of the services of the nursing profession of the state as a whole. The study, therefore, has made an humble attempt to assess the socio–economic conditions of the nurses in the three medical college hospitals of Orissa.

Chapter 2
Profile of Orissa and Medical Colleges in the Sample

Orissa is a State having population of 31,512,070 according to 1991 census. The rate of population growth during the 1981–91 though marginally slower than what it was during 1971–81 decade, is still around 2 per cent per annum which means an addition of 6.33 lakh to the State population annually. The State Government shall have to intensify all its efforts to restrict the annual growth rate to 1.78 per cent as stipulated for the nation. In order to curb the menace of population explosion the State Government is required to strengthen the family planning machinery and at the same time popularise female education. For implementation of the accepted goal of National Health Policy "Health for All by A.D. 2000", a good network of medical institutions with adequate health personnel is required to be developed who would be engaged throughout the State for providing health care to the people. The structural framework for the delivery of health programmes should be so designed so that the health care should not only be available but it has to be accessible and affordable and appropriate to the needs of the people. In this endeavour, the role of nurses to impart immunisation, health education and sanitation is very much necessary.

2.1 Orissa: Socio–economic Profile

Orissa, having vast natural resources and launching a good number of developmental programmes in different plan periods, still stands behind all the States having 56 per cent of its population living below poverty line in 1987–88 according to the estimates of Expert Group appointed by the Planning Commission. The State economy exhibits all the characteristics of under development like growing incidence of poverty, unemployment, low per capita income and inadequate development of infrastructure etc.

Demographic Features

The land area of the State is about 155,707 sq. kms. which is 4.74 per cent of the land area of the country. According to the 1991 census, population of the State stood at 316.60 lakh which is 3.74 per cent of the population of India. The sex ratio, *i.e.*, female per 1000 male witnessed a fall from 981 in 1981 to 971 in 1991. But the density of population is raised from 169 to 203 per sq. km. from 1981 to 1991. Similarly, literacy rate has increased to 49.1 per cent in 1991 as against 34.2 per cent in 1981. The male and female literacy rate in Orissa is 63.1 per cent and 34.7 per cent respectively in 1991 (Economic Survey, 1993–94).

Employment

The unemployment problem is not only a state problem rather a global problem. A bulk of the working force remain without an assured employment as there is no job opportunity both in rural and urban areas either in public or in the private sector. It is estimated that by the end of 1993–94 backlog of unemployment would reach a level of 5.72 lakh. Pressure of population is considerably high on land. Nearly 63.75 per cent of the total working population depends upon agriculture and its allied activities, in spite of various self–employment schemes and wage employment schemes. Out of total working force (32.78 per cent); cultivator constitutes 14.53 per cent, agricultural labour constitute 9.41 per cent, labour in household constitute 1.02 per cent and persons engaged in other activities constitute 7.83 per cent.

Agriculture

Agriculture is the life blood of State economy cropped area has marginally increased by 3.2 per cent in 1992–93 over that of 1991–92. Rice being the staple food of the people of Orissa, it continues to be the leading crop. The area under rice was 42.61 lakh hectares which estimated capacity of earning is 62.20 MT (Economic Survey 1993–94). So far as consumption of fertilisers is concerned, in 1991 Orissa's consumption stands at as low as

21 kg per hectare as compared to its neighbouring states, like Andhra Pradesh 119 kg, West Bengal 90 kg, Bihar 58 kg and Madhya Pradesh 36 kg.

Irrigation

Irrigation is the prime requirement for agriculture to provide a full time employment to agricultural labourers round the year to facilitate multiple cropping. Sustained and systematic programme for development of irrigation facilities has been the core policy of the Government. Out of total irrigation potential created major and medium projects accounts for 45.6 per cent; minor flow 18.2 per cent, minor (lift) 13.2 per cent and other sources 23.0 per cent respectively. To store the run off rain water and improve moisture content of the soil, 7525 water harvesting structures have been constructed by the end of 1992–93 (Economic Survey, 1993–94).

Power

Orissa is a power deficit State. It mainly depends upon Hydro Power Projects and Thermal Power Projects of the State sector. It has to purchase heavy units of power from Central sector as share and from industries like NALCO and Indian Changechrome Ltd. etc. So far as per capita consumption of electricity is concerned the position of Orissa is much below the national level. It is now 226.0 KWH as against the all India average of 330.6 KWH.

Industry

Despite of abundant natural resources and raw materials, Orissa continues to be industrially backward. In the Central Sector large industries like Rourkela Steel Plant, NALCO at Anugul and Damanjodi, Paradeep Phosphate Ltd., Fertiliser plant at Rourkela, Heavy Water Project at Talcher and Carriage Repair Workshop at Bhubneswar were set up prior to 1990 and after that only some countable progress is made in small scale industries sector. For accelerating the pace of industrial growth during the 8th Five Year Plan, the New Industrial Policy of 1992 was announced which offered attractive incentives and provide marketing support for small industrial units and encourage private entrepreneurs of invest in industrial ventures.

Mineral

Orissa is gifted with vast amount of mineral reserve of coal, chromite, iron ore, bauxite and manganese ore, lead ore to the tune of 44304 million tonnes, 183 million tonnes, 3120 million tonnes, 1626 million tonnes, 49 million tonnes and 2.6 million tonnes respectively. But due to lack of proper investment, modernisation and absence of infrastructure facilities, it is not properly exploited.

Education

Economic development of a country is incomplete without development of human resources. However, the different education policy has attained 49 per cent of literacy in the State level. The drop–out rate among the children in the age group of 6–11 in respect of general, SC and ST category of students in 1991 was 46 per cent, 56 per cent and 72 per cent respectively. So State Government has taken positive measures by providing better schooling facilities within each reach, mid–day meals and free boarding and lodging for SC and ST students for retention of children in the school. By the end of 1992–93 the number of Primary schools, M.E. schools and High schools are of the order of 53,756, 11,716 and 4,921 respectively. Number of teachers employed were 117,492, 39,031 and 44,289 in Primary school, M.E. school and High school respectively. For providing higher education, 615 colleges were functioning with intake capacity of 2.99 lakh students, 4 Engineering colleges with intake capacity of 781 students, 11 Engineering schools/Poly techniques with intake capacity of 1155 under Government Management were functioning in the State during 1992–93 (Economic Survey, 1993–94).

Fishery

Orissa is endowed with marine, brackish water and fresh water fishery resources to improve the economic conditions of the State. Per capita fish consumption in Orissa is 4.89 kg. and exported outside is nearly 90.1 lakh MT. State Government have taken up Animal Husbandry and Dairy Development programmes to increase the livestock productivity through adoption of scientific breeding, better feeding and management practices. Significant progress has been made in regard to milk and egg production in the State. But per capita availability is less in comparison to national level. According to 1991 livestock census, the cattle population in Orissa was 135.77 lakh of which the working cattle constituted 45.93 lakh and milk cattle 41.90 lakh. The number of buffaloes, sheep, goats, pigs constituted about 15.09 lakh, 18.41 lakh, 48.04 lakh and

5.90 lakh respectively. For providing animal health care, there were 519 veterinary hospitals with 519 Animal Physicians as on 31st March, 1993.

Science and Technology

Science and technological inputs are essential for economic growth of the State. An outlay of Rs. 7500,00 lakh has been proposed under State plan during 8th Five Year Plan for expenditure on schemes like (a) Non–conventional Sources of Energy, (b) Scientific Research, (c) Integrated Rural Energy Planning Programme, (d) Large and Medium industries. Orissa Renewable Energy Development Agency (OREDA) has taken the responsibility of planning, co–ordinating, monitoring, executing and evaluating the programmes in the State.

Women Status

In spite of constitutional provisions and legislative measures for protection of women rights and welfare, the status of women continues to remain backward due to illiteracy and ignorance. In order to bring them to the main stream, the Department of Women Development and Mahila Vikash Nigam have been established to set up women training centre, widow pension and rehabilitative service to women in distress to raise their status in the society. In 1991, reservation of 30 per cent of seats in all the local bodies to introduce and enjoy equal political rights in the state.

State Income

In the economy of Orissa, agriculture occupies an important place. As this sector contributes more than 50 per cent to the State income. But predominance of this sector creates great deal of instability in the rate of growth of income due to fluctuation in agricultural production depending on weather conditions. Flood, drought, cyclone occur very often causing substantial loss to crop production which brings about fluctuations also. The per capita income of the state which was Rs. 3077 in 1990–91 increased to Rs.3816 in 1991–92 at current prices. The per capita income of 1992–93, as per the quick estimates, at current and constant prices (1980–81) stood at Rs. 3963 and Rs.1442 respectively (Economic Survey, 1993–94).

Population Status

In Orissa according to 1991 census 22.21 per cent are Scheduled Tribe and 16.2 per cent are Scheduled Caste. Their number is 7,032,000 (ST) and 5,129,000 (SC) according to 1991 census. Number of Scheduled Tribes people are more mainly in Mayurbhanj, Sundargarh and Sambalpur in comparison to Ganjam, Puri and Cuttack. Similarly number of Scheduled Castes people are more in Cuttack, Ganjam and Puri.

2.2 Profile of Medical Institutes in Orissa

The aim and objective of National Health Policy is to provide health services for the unprivileged and under–privileged groups and rural population through a network of medical institutes, such as hospitals, dispensaries, PHCs and Additional PHCs located through –out the State both in rural and urban areas. Table 1 depicts the expansion of medical institutes in the State from the year 1989–90 to 1992–93.

Table 1: Number of Medical Institutes functioning in Orissa

Position as on	*hospitals*	*Community Health Centres*	*Dispensaries*	*PHCs*	*Additional PHCs*
1	*2*	*3*	*4*	*5*	*6*
31.3.90	181	50	140	261	612
31.3.91	181	75	140	261	612
31.3.92	176	110	145	235	626
31.3.93	176	110	139	232	626

Source : Director of Health Services, Government of Orissa, Bhubneswar.

Due to conversion of hospitals and dispensaries to Additional PHCs and Community Health Centres, the number of hospitals, dispensaries and PHCs have decreased. Upto 1983, 1283 medical institutes were functioning and providing health care to the people. The number of hospital bed has been increased from 52 per lakh populations, to 53 per lakh populations.

Besides those allopathic medical institutions there are large number of Homeopathic Institutions and Ayurvedic Institutions are functioning throughout the state. Table 2 and 3 show the details of those institutions.

Table 2 : Homoeopathic Institutions, Patients treated in it and Beds available in Orissa

Year	*hospitals (Nos.)*	*Dispensaries (Nos.)*	*Beds available (Nos.)*	*Doctors/ Nurses (Nos.)*	*Homeo Assistants or Nurses (Nos.)*	*Patients treated ('000 Nos.)*
1	*2*	*3*	*4*	*5*	*6*	*7*
1987	7	321	206	365	352	61,57
1988	7	321	206	366	353	58,90
1989	7	346	166	368	361	62,79
1990	6	382	150	414	394	68,26
1991	6	442	165	477	495	68,65

Source : Director, Indian Medicine and Homoeopath Principals of different Homoeopathic and Ayurvedic colleges in Orissa.

Table 3 : Ayurvedic Institutions, Patients treated in it and Beds available in Orissa

Year	*hospitals (Nos.)*	*Dispensaries (Nos.)*	*Beds available (Nos.)*	*Doctors/ (Kaviraj) (Nos.)*	*Nurses (Nos.)*	*Patients ('000 Nos.)*
1	*2*	*3*	*4*	*5*	*6*	*7*
1987	8	387	295	442	16	44,59
1988	8	387	295	445	16	44,45
1989	10	412	318	470	23	45,18
1990	9	452	273	491	21	47,41
1991	9	499	284	541	23	50,60

N.B. : Except Berhampur Ayurvedic college (Ankuspur, Ganjam) for the year 1990 and 1991.

Source : Director, Indian Medicine and Homoeopath Principals of different Homoeopathic and Ayurvedic colleges in Orissa.

medical institutions are not evenly distributed throughout the districts of the state. There is inter regional disparities in the establishment of medical institutions (Table 4).

Table 4 : District–wise (undivided) number of Medical Institutions in Orissa as on 31st March, 1993

District	*Hospi-tals*	*Dispen-saries*	*PHC*	*Addl. PHC*	*medical Aid Centre*	*Subsi-diary Health Centre*	*Comm-unity Health Centre*	*Mobile Health Centre*
1	*2*	*3*	*4*	*5*	*6*	*7*	*8*	*9*
Balasore	8	19	12	47	5	22	9	–
Bolangir	9	4	13	29	3	5	8	–
Cuttack	23	25	32	108	8	23	10	–
Dhenkanal	12	7	13	32	2	8	7	1
Ganjam	17	19	25	51	2	10	7	2
Kalahandi	10	4	15	30	1	8	5	9
Keonjhar	10	4	7	37	2	10	8	3
Koraput	16	14	27	79	1	20	17	7
Mayurbhanj	11	5	16	44	2	15	12	2
Phulbani	10	6	13	27	2	4	3	2
Puri	29	23	24	55	4	23	6	–
Sambalpur	12	6	23	55	3	15	12	–
Sundargarh	9	3	12	32	3	9	6	1
Orissa	176	139	232	626	38	172	110	27

Source : Directorate of Health Services, Government of Orissa, Bhubneswar.

Besides these institutions the team to provide health care system in the state, there is nursing community. There are large number of nursing schools to train them and one nursing college at Berhampur is established to provide them higher education in the state. There are three nursing schools at three medical college hospitals such as SCB Medical College, Cuttack, VSS Medical College, Burla and MKCG Medical College, Berhampur where Chief–Matron is the nursing executive head.

Orissa, the poorest and least developed State after Bihar, had always been deprived of the best medicare facilities. Existing facilities were nowhere near the best and with shortage of funds along with faulty planning and networking made things worse. During all these years patients were exposed to the poor existing services and they never demanded more as there was no bench marking. Only the neo rich had the privilege of visiting hospitals outside the state. Orissa had three medical colleges for caring 4 crores of population. Hence, there are always fewer beds than the demand. At times there are no doctors, nurses and no proper equipment. Out of necessity, the middle class patient had to depend on the private nursing homes or had to visit outside the state and spend his entire savings. Be it an advanced general procedure or a super specialty tertiary care with all ultra modern facilities, Orissa has them all.

In spite of the fact that the doctors, technicians, and the nurses are not demi Gods nor can they perform any miracles, they work round the clock to save the life of the patients. Health, which used to have the least priority, is getting its due importance. With changing life style, irregular food habits, high–pressure job, life will certainly invite all kinds of diseases. Hence, there shall be a demand for health care facilities. Orissa, has to keep pace with this.

Chapter 3
Socio–economic Characteristics of Nurses in Orissa

3.1 Introduction

The traditional concept of a women's role in the economic life of our country has undergone a revolutionary change in the present century. Previously women was not regarded as a "worker" who produced " marketable goods". She was at the most graded as a secondary worker – a labour reserve compressed into a relatively narrow range of low income, low skilled jobs or eased out of labour force in a male dominated world. Because culturally little girls are tought or they learn from their mothers or the relatives that their decision making capacity is limited, the boys can do it better; with the result that her decision making capacity gets stunned. Often she remains grateful for what she has been given and cannot think of negotiating for anything more. But with the rising tempo of industrialisation in the country and consequent development of trade, commerce, social and commercial services, more and more women started accepting paid employment. There has been a significant increase in women's employment in various fields such as education, research, public administration, firms and factories etc. The number of women workers has specially increased in the tertiary sector of the economy.

Similarly, a large percentage of women workers in the country is employed in the nursing profession. A women is a loving mother and by nature she is kind, patient and sympathetic. Whenever she sees an ailing person, she visualises a helpless child in him/her and voluntarily comes forward to nurse him/her. Nursing, in fact, is a noble profession where a nurse serves the patients consciously, help them to get rid of pains and strains and pulls them back to life from the clutches of death. The nurse is like an angel for the patient. This has been a tradition night from Florence Nightingale who served the dying and the wounded soldiers in the Cremean battle field. The "Lady with the lamp" unmindful of her own life and health attended the wounded soldiers to give them whatever she could and carried on her mission day and night risking her even life in the battle field. Every nurse who nurses a patient with care, love and tenderness forgetting even her hunger and thirst gives him prompt and accurate medical care, feels an inner satisfaction and an external joy when the same dying patient comes back to life. Only a blood relation could act and feel like that. That is why a nurse is called "Sister". She is proud of her profession because the word "Nurse" represents the following qualities in her; 'N' stands for nobility of the profession and the family of a nurse; 'U' stands for unity among all nurses; 'R' stands for regularity in work; 'S' stands for sympathy for the patients and 'E' stands for excellent etiquettes. A lady is eminently suited for this job of noble thought and wises because of her inner flow of love, affection and compassion.

3.2 Socio–economic Status

Different variables have been used to delineate a status structure. The two most common measures used to stratify a population have been those of prestige rating of person and the socio–economic status scales. The most commonly used status scales are income, education and occupation. Both individual income and educational attainment which are used as measure of socio–economic status are known to be correlated with occupational ranks and both can be taken as aspects of occupational status. Education is a basis for entry into many occupations from which most people drive their income. "Education is a very large factor in the social status of the workers and wages or salary income is a very large factor in their economic status". Students of Sociology are of the view that the social status of a family is more likely to reflect the occupation of the husband than that of the wife, if both are employed.

The usual operational indicators of social status, particularly income and education are subjectively seen as more important elements than the prestige status of an occupation in a social structure. There is a slippery distinction between social status and economic status, because there is both a functional nexus and a temporal order in the relationship of occupation to education. But income and occupation are functionally related. We have, therefore, the following sequence : a man qualifies himself for occupational life by obtaining an education; as a consequence of pursuing his occupation, he obtains income. Occupation, therefore, is the intervening activity linking income to education. Characterising an occupation according to prevailing levels of education and income of its incumbents, "we are not only estimating its social and economic status, but also describing one of its major cause and one its major effects".

Status Images

Rural people identify several factors responsible to put an individual in the upper level of society. These are income, leadership, polished behaviour, character and responsibility. Income alone is not over empahsised. Similarly, urban people put forth several criteria, such as, income, education, one's achievement in a special field, social service and good character to place a person either in the high or low status group. Criteria used to identify the persons in the middle group are moderate education and income rather than one's caste.

Subjective assessment of status is necessary because of following reasons:

1. It may provide an insight into the criteria which people use to make social divisions in society.
2. It may locate new classes, castes and sub–culture etc. which are on the move.
3. It may trace the perceived barriers as channels of social mobility.
4. It may reveal the frictions and conflicts between different social layers.

The criteria used to identify the person's status are income, leadership, behaviour, character and respectability. Some studies have been made to determine the criteria of socio–economic status which combine several criteria such as income, one's education in a special field, social service and good character to place a person either in the higher or lower status category. But some believe that "a person is expected to build–up hope for a better future world by accumulating merits. it could also help him to get born to a better caste in the next world".

The variables that determine the social status in a changing life pattern are caste, character, dress, education, food, housing, income, neighbourhood, recreation, social service and mode of transport. A study fixes the rank of several variables in determining social status (Table 5).

Table 5: Mean Rank of Status Criteria expressed by Rural and Urban Informants

Rural	*Mean Rank*	*Urban–Industrial*
Education	1	Education
Character	2	Social Service
Social Service	3	Character
Income	4	Income
Caste	5	Housing
Housing	6	Neighbourhood
Neighbourhood	7	Caste
Dress	8	Dress
Food	9	Food
Mode of Transport	10	Recreation
Recreation	11	Mode of Transport

Source : Bopegamage, A. and Veeraraghaban, P.V., Status Images in Changing India. Australia and New Zealand Book Co. Pvt. Ltd., 12, Thomas Street, Chatswood, N.S.W., 1977.

A set of qualities is also ranked according to the degree of importance indicating their weight in determining social status. The qualities are caste, courage, cunningness, education, honesty, intelligence, the money stock and the social contact. By this method, the mean rank order of qualities stands for the two samples, rural and urban–industrial (Table 6).

Table 6 : The Mean Rank of Qualities needed to rise in status

Rural	*Mean Rank*	*Urban–Industrial*
Education	1	Education
Intelligence	2	Intelligence
Honesty	3	Honestey
Money	4	Perserverance
Caste	5	Money
Cunningness	6	Whom you know
Whom you know	7	Courage
Courage	8	Cunningness
Perseverance	9	Caste

Source : Bopegamage, A. and Veeraraghaban, P.V., Status Images in Changing India. Australia and New Zealand Book Co. Pvt. Ltd., 12, Thomas Street, Chatswood, N.S.W., 1977.

The study concludes that education is the single most important factor to raise the socio–economic status of any person because both in the rural and urban areas, the highest premium is attached to this factor.

For finer discrimination self replacement in the status hierarchy a "**seven step**" ladder has been used. The top step represents the highest status and the step at the bottom the lowest (Fig. 2).

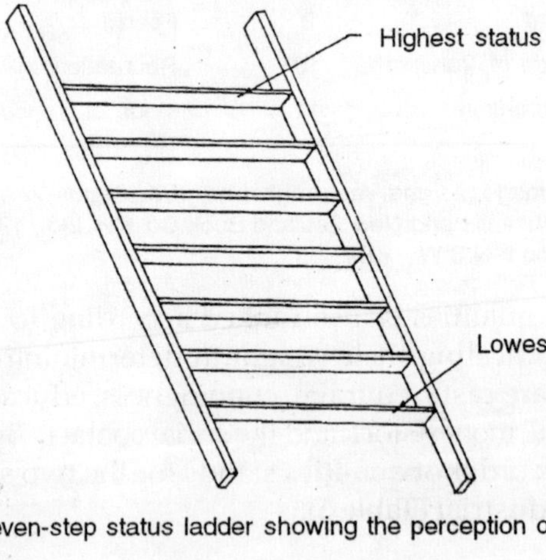

Fig. 2: seven-step status ladder showing the perception of status.

The Social System and Nurses

People work in all kinds of organisation. Organisations are social systems which represents a complex set of human relationship with limitless interaction within the groups and sub–groups. If one wishes to work in organisations or to manage them, it is necessary to understand their operation. Organisations combine society and people, – technology and humanity. Technology is difficult, but when people are added to it we get an immensely complex social system that almost defies understanding. However, society must form organisations and use them well because they are necessary to achieve the benefits. Modern society depends on organisations for its survival. Human behaviour in organisations arises from people's deep–seated needs and value systems. There is no idealistic solution to organisational problems. All that can be done is to increase our understanding and skill so that human relationships at work would improve. The social system has significant bearing on the job. It influences the attitude of the worker and sets a value for the particular work. People, therefore, can be made to work effectively if they are prepared to think about themselves in human terms.

All organisations operate within an external environment. A single organisation does not exist alone. It is part of a larger system that contains thousands of other elements. All these mutually influence one another in a complex system that becomes the life style of the people. The external environment influences the attitudes of the people, affects their working conditions and provides opportunities to attain fulfilment. Just as people have psychological needs, they also have social roles and status. Their behaviour is influenced by status. The organisational environment is a dynamic change rather than a static set of relations. Nurses learn to depend on their culture which gives them stability and security. If there is cultural shock in life and a feeling of confusion, insecurity, it may bring chaos and confusion in the nursing community. Viewed from this angle, the social system is very important to determine the behaviour of the nursing personnel and it is in this context that a discussion of traditional and modern approach to the problem is felt necessary.

The traditional concept of a woman's role in the economic life of our country has undergone a revolutionary change in the present century. Previously women was not regarded as a **"worker"** who produced **"marketable goods"**. She was at the most graded as a secondary worker – a labour reserve compressed into a relatively narrow range of low income, low skilled jobs or eased out of labour force in a male dominated world. Because culturally little girls are taught or they learn from their mothers or the environment that their decision making capacity is limited, the boys can do it better; with the result that her decision making capacity gets stunned. Often she remains grateful for what she has been given and can not think of negotiating for anything more. But with the rising tempo of industrialisation in the country and the consequent development of trade, commerce, social and commercial services, more and more women started accepting paid employment. The condition today is that since the year 1901 there has been a significant increase in women's employment in various fields such as education, research, public administration, firms and factories etc. The number of women workers has specially increased in the tertiary sector of the economy.

Similarly, a large percentage of women workers in the country is employed in the nursing profession. A women is a loving mother and by nature she is kind, patient and sympathetic. Whenever she sees an ailing person, she visualises a helpless child in him/her and voluntarily comes forward to nurse him/her. Nursing, in fact, is a noble profession where a nurse serves the patients consciously, helps them to get rid of pains and strains and pulls them back to life from the clutches of death. The nurse is like an angel for the patient. This has been a tradition right from Florence Nightingale who served the dying and the wounded soldiers in the Cremean battle field. The **"Lady with the lamp"** unmindful of her own life and health attended the wounded soldiers to give them whatever she could and carried on her mission day and night risking her own life in the battle field. Every nurse who nurses a patient with care, love and tenderness forgetting even her hunger and thirst gives him prompt and accurate medical care, feels an inner satisfaction and an external joy when the same dying patient comes back to life. Only a blood relation could act and feel like that. That is why a nurse is called **"Sister"**. She is proud of her profession because the word "**Nurse**" represents the following qualities in her; '**N**' stands for nobility of the profession and the family of a nurse; '**U**' stands for unity among all nurses; '**R**' stands for regularity in work; 'S' stands for sympathy for the patients and 'E' stands for excellent etiquettes. A lady is eminently suited for this job of noble thought and wises because of her inner flow of love, affection and compassion.

Society sometimes does not duly recognise the invaluable services of nurses. There is a feeling that they serve out of economic necessity. One has to serve to earn one's bread. But in case of the nurses, it is not a question of bread and butter alone. It transcends beyond that mundane consideration and goes to a higher plane of service and sacrifice. Some criticise the nature of nursing services and underestimate it. The general attitude towards the job sometimes demoralises the nurses and on the other hand, they do not receive so attractive salary to compensate this loss of face and low wages, over duty and not very congenial social attitudes and these are the real hurdles before the nursing community. Demoralisation of the community and loss of recognition have left a deep scar on the cadre of the profession. Man does not live by bread alone. He needs job satisfaction status, recognition, cooperation from colleagues, mutual understanding, trust and confidence from superiors and subordinates. He also needs opportunities to test and display his skill and needs appreciation. He is also conscious of his image and dignity. In short, the nurse needs no lip service alone but is in need of prestige, status and reasonable economic compensation for her sacrifice to lead a dignified life in a grossly materialistic world.

Nurse versus Doctor

Nursing today is regarding as the sheet anchor of our total health care delivery system and nursing personnel form a major part of the health care manpower. It is imperative for the nursing personnel to improve their skill in management, supervision, research and evaluation for a successful deliverance of the health care system. Kharpade echoes the same sentiment when she says that the concept of nursing brings to our mind the image of **"The lady with the lamp — Florence Nightingale"**. This concept has expanded over the years and it is not longer confined to hospitals and patients' care alone. It may also remind all nurses that like most worthwhile things of life, nursing was also born out of strainous struggle and hardship. The pioneers in nursing profession have withstood tremendous pressure and resistance and brought not only acceptance but recognition to the present concept of nursing. Today, the nurses are an important link in our total health care delivery system. No medical team is complete without nurses. Apart from assisting the doctor, a nurse has to play an important role in her own right in health care. The theme, **"Health for all–All for Health"** is the nurses' concern. Their mission is to provide, as far as practicable, primary health care, including preventive, promotive and rehabilitative service at the door steps of the people. They may emerge to be the most important of the changing agents in the value system of the community by virtue of being the closest to it. They help in bringing down maternal mortality rate, enhance the rate of survival, promote acceptance of family welfare practices and improve health and hygiene awareness. In all probability, their status and position will enthuse them for greater dedication and sacrifice which will ultimately benefit the country and society.

The Mohite Committee Report rightly points out that next to doctor, nurse is the most important member of the health team. Whether in a hospital or in the field, it is skills, attitude, competence, confidence and morale that largely determine the quality and standard of health care and medical care offered by the services to the community. Today the importance of health care has increased tremendously. medical Science is fast advancing and scientists have been able to conquer completely or nearly so many of the communicable diseases like smallpox but many new disease have appeared. In the developing countries like India, conditions are much worse. Problems like family planning have to be tackled with great care with due consideration to its various related aspects. Moreover, lack of scientific attitude is another matter of concern. These countries want quick urbanisation and industrial growth without realising the danger of pollution and other concomitant problems. All these have complicated the problem of today's health care system to such an extent that the entire technique of health care has radically changed to meet the requirements of the people adequately. The new progressive techniques are curative, preventive and health promotive activities. In the light of these developments, the nursing profession assumes tremendous importance and has become an indispensable part of the entire health planning of the nation.

Nurse is an important link between the doctor and the patient. She is a crucial element in transmitting the elementary idea of health, hygiene and family welfare. In view of the growing importance of this key element in the health team, improvement in the curriculum, and organisation, advancement in the techniques of training and teaching and development of new approaches to the profession as a whole are necessary. Those who choose nursing as a career should be adequately equipped to participate effectively in the programmes of health promotion and the Health Care Delivery System, so as to enable them to enter into the 21st Century with confidence and meet the targets of **"Health for All by 2000 AD"**.

Though the importance and vital contribution of nurses in the health–care system can never be defined and their services constitute an essential element in the medical world, no separate allotments are made in the budget for Nursing and para–nursing development. The entire budget is classified under medical Education and Training and a separate allotment is given to encourage Indian Medicine. Since the planners are medical professionals and the bureaucrats are influenced by the former, almost the entire budget is spent on medical and para–medical education procuring expensive and sophisticated equipment and drugs for medical diagnosis or treatment and little is left for nursing which is considered to be just one of the para–medical branches. Same is the story for sanction of posts in Nursing at all levels especially in hospitals where no educated nurse wishes to work. In advanced countries there are two most important heads under which budget allotment is made. The first is medical and para–medical consisting of doctors, technicians, technologists, dieticians, physiotherapists, occupational therapists etc. and the second is Nursing and para–nursing consisting of nurses, midwives, health visitors, practical auxiliary nurses, aides, house keepers, catering staff, sanitation staff, messengers, receptionists etc. Besides general education in nursing at different levels, additional training is given to nurses in specialised areas to cater to the hospital and community needs.

Nursing is vital for the nation's health. There is a saying that, "God made mother because He could not be present every where at all times". In the same way the health system created a professional called a nurse (Like a mother who has to be a female) because a doctor may not remain present everywhere at all times. Nurses have multifarious roles at the Central and State level. By virtue of their training in midwifery and paediatric nursing where she gets knowledge of growth, development, psychology, sociology and planned parenthood and skills of caring for the mother during antenatal, delivery, post–natal and carrying for the child–newborn, toddler, pre–school, school and adolescent, she has the ability to promote medical care and prevent disease to the mother and child and motivate the parents towards planned parenthood.

Nurses' teaching of personal hygiene, sanitation, nutrition, cooking and first–aid are also very important. To change the habits and attitude towards health care and to promote health awareness is a time consuming process which does not work merely by achieving targets of immunisation. A lot of motivational work has to be done, hence knowledge of psychology and sociology is essential to understand the behavioural dynamics which needs to be changed to reach the destination. Similarly, the nurse acts as an angel of mercy. People under stress and sickness require constant attention of a kind, skilful, resourceful and tactful persons, who could mitigate the fear of the unknown, classifies doubts and explains and supports medical procedure. The nurse like an **Angel of Mercy** performs these essential and invaluable tasks in the hospitals and brings solace and hope to the millions of mankind.

Nurses play an active role in the filed of school healths. She is a mother to the children, peer to the teachers and a friend to the parents. Health education, health check–up, teaching of first–aid, home nursing, mothercraft, family planning, counselling the teachers and parents are some of the functions of school health nurse who is on the school staff. Besides, she assists the children during annual medical check–up. Nurses make significant contribution in the filed of family planning and family welfare. Normally a women likes to confide fears, doubts and ignorance in another female specially in matters relating to marital and children's problem. Offering self with frequent home visit gives confidence to the women and trust is built. Thus, any targets of family planning or immunisation and others can be met better in the long run. Working with the family with complexity of personality profiles at the varied age level in assisting to help themselves is not difficult but time consuming which requires emotional maturity and sound knowledge and skills of the nurse.

A nurse utilising her technical skill of nursing to assist a handicap person has to be an ego booster to strengthen the self image of the person who is due for rehabilitation. Somato–psychic nursing is a speciality by itself where a nurse is an expert in psycho–social and physical therapies. It can be for variety of handicaps classified under orthopaedic neurological, leprosy, medical visual, audio, speech, mentally sub–normal etc. Relatives or family or work places are equally important in the rehabilitation process, although for every nurse the rehabilitation starts from the day he reports sick or injured.

As the services to people are expanding, her role becomes more and more pronounced. In the modern times the nurse may be a public relation officer, co–ordinator and collaborator. She is a public functionary who has the maximum contact with people under stress and their relatives. Besides getting good recruits for nursing, she also conveys good will of the government to the people and people's needs to the government. She provides a healthy link between people and authorities of the centre, Institute, State of Centre. Further, in the hospital one patient may be visited by ten other members of the health team and they may leave with order but it is the nursing team which coordinates these orders for the best benefit of the patient. Collaboration will only be possible when the nursing team also is equally qualified in number to present their observation and suggestion on the treatment required. Collaborative decisions are always more fruitful and invite more cooperation.

The current world situation is such that a nurse may get involved in innumerable circumstances requiring action on her part to safeguard human rights in different situations. Conflicting situations are also on the rise including internal political upheaval, strife or internecine war. The action of nurses to safeguard human rights is not restricted only in times of political upheaval and war. It can also arise in prisons or in the normal work situation of any nurse where abuse of patients, nurses or others is witnessed or suspected. Nurses have a responsibility in each of these situations to take action to safeguard the rights of those involved.

In the field of preservation and improvement of the human environment nurses' role is very vital. This vast and urgent task may be possible by the joint effort of nurses and every professional.

The nurses' role is to detect ill effects of the environment on the human health and vice verse, apply knowledge in the routine business, inform preventive measures about health hazards, collaborate with health authorities pointing out health care aspects of environment and health hazards and assist communities in their action on environmental health problems.

Nursing as a profession will have to accept responsibility for significant functions and develop abilities to prescribe preventive, curative and rehabilitative treatment in a responsible and accountable way. They play their role in the struggle to remove obstacles in the path of better access to basic health care.

Nurses may be expected to assume a major role in the implementation of primary health care strategies. It includes such functions as training primary health care workers, establishing educational programmes for health workers, helping communities to identify their needs and working as referral agents, managers and team leaders. These activities require new skills and motivation on the part of the nurse which must be acquired. Simultaneously, forces outside nursing education can bring about changes; such as (i) changes in government policy, (ii) redefinition of role and function of nurse, (iii) community needs. Expected success depends upon simultaneous interaction of all forces (Fig. 3).

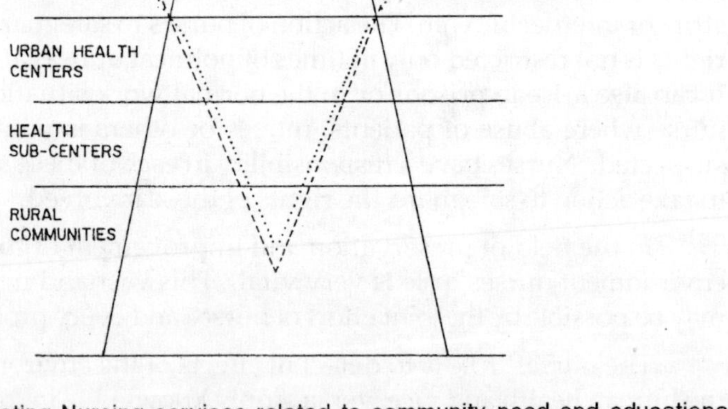

Fig. 3: Existing Nursing services related to community need and educational experiences.

Building the nation's health is, in the final analysis, a collective responsibility and the importance of team work in this sphere can never be underestimated. The whole idea has been summarised in the following verse :

> "Some one has blended the plaster
>
> some one has carried the store
>
> neither the man nor the master
>
> ever has builded alone
>
> only by working together
>
> things are accomplished by man
>
> all have a share in the beauty
>
> all have a part in the plan."

Nurse is an important partner in the medical team. Her multifarious roles as a mother, angel of mercy, watch–dog in an industry, ego booster for physical handicaps, coordinator, safeguarder of human rights, preserver of human environment and primary health care has made her an indispensable link in the complete chain of the health care system.

The Other Side

The peculiarities of the occupation make the profession both interesting and challenging. The profession is dominated by women. It is observed that almost all the employees in the nursing staff in any hospital are women. Most of them are from lower middle class families and accept the job on economic compulsions. The married among them in addition to hospital duties have to shoulder responsibilities at home like cooking, household work and looking after children etc. Others are also not free from domestic work in a traditional society. Since they are from the low income group they cannot afford the luxury of domestic servants to run the households. They have to do all work by themselves and that naturally put tremendous strain on them. The nature of the profession keeps the duty hours totally different from the official duty hours.

A nurse on duty during day time has to reach her work–place as early as 7.30 am in the morning to be relieved at about 2.30 pm. Moreover, she has to keep a margin of an hour or so for travelling to and from the work–place. Duty hours always change according to the changing needs of the hospital. A nurse has to do night duty, overtime and emergency duty which other employees are not called upon to do in their services. Nursing presupposes a humanitarian outlook, a sense of service and sacrifice and a total commitment to work. Devoid of these qualities, the profession loses its meaning and essence.

Teaching and nursing are the two main professions where most of the educated women are engaged not only in India but also in other parts of the world. Every mother is a loving nurse, the only difference being a mother looks after her own children, husband and her most near and dear ones without remuneration. A nurse, on the other hand, has to sacrifice her own comfort of home and family life to look after the known and the unknown irrespective of caste, creed, religion or language with the expectation of a monetary reward. In short, she is said to have been doing something "**to cure sometimes, to relieve often but to comfort always**". But she very often feels professionally neglected, economically depressed and socially underestimated. People with a narrow vision attribute many of the ills of the present day medical system to the malfunctioning and deterioration in the nursing care only. It may be partly correct but certainly not the whole truth. The poor economic scenario is the prime factor for the deterioration of the quality care. Some of the important aspects of the problem are : Work load, pay scale, income sources, incentives and job prospects, expenditure pattern and saving and investment.

Work Load

In modern times work load is a status issue. More physical strain with less leisure is a symbol of poor economic status. The study reveals that 99 per cent of the nurses are said to have estimates their workload quite in excess of their normal load. Only one per cent has viewed it as "just" either because of their innocence and ignorance about the correct position or because of some other extraneous reasons. Their union (ONEA), therefore, is legitimately demanding for overtime payment. The recommended number of nurses by INC is three beds for one nurse (1:3) for teaching institutions (Medial college hospitals) and 5 beds for a nurse (1:5) for non–teaching institutions. The following example is a case in point which illustrates the reality and proves that each nurse has to work for 30 beds (Fig. 4).

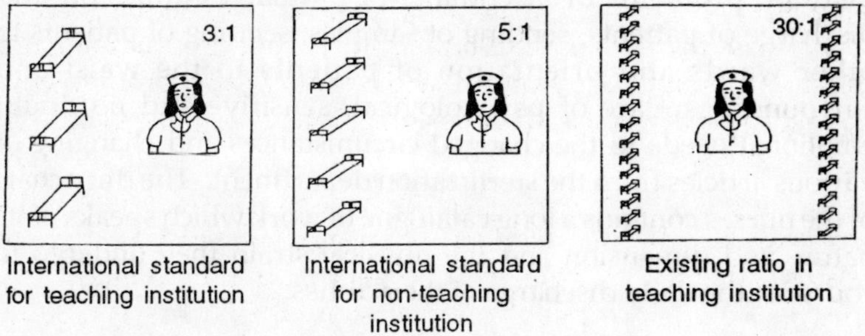
3:1
5:1
30:1
International standard for teaching institution
International standard for non-teaching institution
Existing ratio in teaching institution

Fig. 4: Nurse – Bed Ratio.

In the SCB Medical College hospital the number of beds in the TB ward is 60 and the average occupancy at any point of time is 55. The number of staff nurses posted in the ward is eight which falls far short of the INC standard of 20. The nurses have an 8 hours shift pattern. Out of eight, one is always usually absent due to casual leave, maternity leave or off duty. Out of the effective strength of seven staff nurses one is kept in charge of medicine in the ward and two each in the morning, evening and night shifts respectively are posted on duty.

An honest and proper handling and taking over of charge by nurses during the change in shifts would take at least 4 minutes per patient, the process of recording the temperature would take minimum three minutes and recording of blood pressure and pulses would take another two minutes respectively. A simple calculation on the basis of the norm brings the total time required for 55 patients to 33 hrs. and 40 minutes. But they have 24 hours in their hand and in all the three shifts. This proves that the nurses are forced to work for much longer than eight hours without any compensatory allowances or incentives which amounts to economic exploitation.

Besides, the staff nurses have to do certain jobs which basically do not fall under their domain. These jobs are : charting of drugs, distribution of drugs, giving injections, sponging and mouth care, bowel, bladder and back care, taking of samples, suction secretions from the throat, Ryle's tube aspiration, care of i/v drips, making of diet lists, bedding, supervision of electricity, water and other matters, problems of attendants of patients, admission and discharge of patients, sending of samples, sending of patients to other wards and orientation of patients to the ward and surroundings, care of psychological, sensitive and no doubt emotional needs to the changed circumstances and changing of various articles from the sterilization department. The duty chart of the nurses contains a long catalogue of work which speaks of its nature and dimension and the physical strain they undergo in course of the daily discharge of their duties.

Pay Scale

Educational qualification, duration of training, the nature of the job and the degree of risk and responsibility are some of the prime determinants of the pay scales. Viewed from the angles of all these parameters it may be conclusively said that nursing is no way inferior to the services of Junior Engineer when compared on the basis of qualification and experience and is in no way less hazardous and risky than that of a military nursing personnel in the field of his work. But there is a significant difference between the pay scales of nursing personnel in college hospitals and defence services. Similarly, the difference is equally glaring between the pay scale of nurses and that of the Junior Engineers. Difference in their pay scale and promotional opportunities is delineated in Table 7.

A staff nurse with the completion of a three year diploma course draws a basic pay of Rs.4500 in the scale of Rs.4500–7000 whereas a Junior Engineer with a three year diploma is allowed a basic salary of Rs.6500 in the scale of Rs. 6500–9900. Similarly, when a Nursing sister/Assistant Matron after 20–25 years of service reaches the scale of Rs. 4750–8000, a Junior Engineers with completion of only 8 years of service gets a promotion to the rank of Assistant Engineer and ends up with a scale of Rs.6500–10500. A Nursing Sister after 15–20 years of service gets the promotion to the post of Assistant Nursing Superintendent and if changes favour she may be promoted to the post of Deputy Superintendent/Chief Matron and to the next higher rank of Nursing Superintendent.

Table 7: Inter Job Comparison in Orissa (Nurses vs. Junior Engineers)

Rank		*Designation*		*Years of Experience (in years)*		*Normal percentage of promotion*		*Pay Scales*	
1		*2*		*3*		*4*		*5*	
N	*E*	*N*	*E*	*N*	*E*	*N*	*E*	*N*	*E*
1	1	Staff Nurse	Junior Engineer	–	–	–	–	(Rs.1350–2200) Rs.4500–7000	(Rs.1400–2600) Rs.6500–9900
2	2	Nursing Sister/ Assistant Matron	Assistant Engineer	20-25	8-10	10%	25%	(Rs.1400–2300) Rs.4750–8000	(Rs.2000–3500) Rs.6500–10500
3	3	Assistant Nursing Supdt./ Matron	Executive Engineer	15-20 (As Nursing Sister)	8-10 (As Assistant Engineer)	2%	25%	(Rs.1600–2600) Rs.5300–8300	(Rs.3000–4500) Rs.9350–14550
4	4	Deputy Nursing Supdt./ Matron	Superintending Engineer	No fixed years	8-10 (As Executive Engineer)	1%	25%	(Rs.2000–3500) Rs.6500–10500	(Rs.3700–5000) Rs.10650–15850
5	5	Nursing Supdt./ Principal	Chief Engineer	No fixed years	No fixed years	Negligible	10%	(Rs.2000–4000) Rs.8000–13500	(Rs.4800–6300) Rs.12000–16500

N.B. 1. N – Nurses, 2. E – Engineers.

Source: Directorate of Health and Family Welfare, Government of Orissa.

* Figures in the parentheses indicate the pre-revised scale, 1986.

But reaching the last two stages is a rare phenomenon. A look at Table 7 reveals that not only in respect of pay scale but also changes of promotion and prospects are better and brighter in case of the Junior Engineer. The difference in scale of pay between the nurses in the college hospitals and in defence services is also revealing (Table 8).

Table 8: Pay Scale of Military Nursing Service (Pre-revised)

Sl.no.	*Designation*	*Pay Scale*
1.	Lieutenant	Rs. 2000–60–2480
2.	Captain	Rs. 2550–75–3150
3.	Major	Rs. 3200–100–3600
4.	Lt. Colonel	Rs. 3800–100–4100
5.	Colonel	Rs. 4200–100–4400
6.	Brigadier	Rs. 4500–100–4800
7.	Major General	Rs. 4900–100–5200
8.	Local Officers of the Military Nursing Service	Rs. 1640–60–2600–EB–75–2900.

Source: Indian Nursing Year Book, 1989.

Nurses, whether in defence or in medical college hospitals, have to take the risk of life and death. Although same pay is justified for the same work, it is noticed that the scale of nursing personnel in the defence department is pretty high from that of the nursing personnel of medical college hospitals of Orissa as well as of other States. In comparison to other States like Karnataka, Maharashtra, Uttar Pradesh, Delhi as well as Central Government, the scale of pay is better than State of Orissa (Table 9).

Incentives and Job Prospects

One of the important elements in the technical efficiency of any work is the attitude of mind and the readiness to exercise their faculties to the full of the manual working staff. When machines are set to work their performance depends on the will of others and there is no problem of incentive or inducement to work so far as they are concerned. But with human beings the case is quite different. Work by them is not a one dimensional entity, but has intensity as well as duration. Hence the same number of hours

Table 9: Scale of Pay (Rs.) of Nursing Personnel in Centre and Different States (Pre-revised)

Sl. No.	*Designation*	*Centre*	*Orissa*	*Karnataka*	*Andhra Pradesh*	*Maharashtra*	*Uttar Pradesh*	*Delhi*
1.	Staff Nurse	1400-2600	1350-2200	1400-2750	1150-2110	1400-2600	1400-2600	1400-2600
2.	Nursing Sister/ Nursing Supervisor/ Assistant Matron	1640-3500	1400-2300	1600-2900	1280-2440	1640-2900	1600-2900	1640-2900
3.	Assistant Nursing Supdt./Matron	2000-3200	1600-2600	1720-3170	1330-2630	2000-3200	2000-3200	2000-3200
4.	Chief Matron/ Nursing Supdt. Grade-I/ Deputy Nursing Supdt.	2000-3500	2000-3500	2000-3750	1810-3230	2000-3500	2000-3500	2000-3500
5.	Nursing Supdt./ Principal Tutor/ Principal	2200-4000	2200-4000	–	–	2200-4000	2200-4000	2200-4000
6.	ANM/Non-resident Nurse	1200-1800	940-1660	–	–	1200-2040	–	–

Source: Directorate of Health and Family Welfare, Government of Orissa.

worked by the same people may yield a much larger or a much smaller product according as the surrounding and situation leads these people to work at full or at half pressure. Plainly, the incentives to energy that the work is able to provide must play an important part. Under any system except one of dragooned coercion the principles on which wages are regulated largely determine the energy output of the workers and so the general level of productivity. Economic incentives may be both positive and negative. Positive incentives are chances of promotion and prospects and negative incentives are chances of demotion and dismissal. We may call the latter economic disincentive rather. For example, people dealing with retail sales get commission and top manager may have stock options, bonuses and profit sharing. Thus, wage incentive can successfully bring psychological and economic reward. Sometimes long–run incentives are more impressive than short–run one. But there is no such long–run or short–run incentive in any form in the nursing profession of Orissa. Nurses, therefore, do not get any psychological and economic reward for their services.

Incentives and job prospects are two inter related terms which depend upon the factors like promotional opportunities and other internal and external advantages. Those advantages of the nursing profession are uniform allowance, washing allowance, nursing allowance, messing allowance, special pay for special ward, ICU special allowance, Mental hospital special allowance, allowance for night duty, ESIS allowance, ration allowance, house rent, stitching allowances, non–practicing allowance and compensatory salary etc.

The avenues of promotion for the nursing personnel are extremely limited. To be more precise, it is hardly one per cent as compared to the much higher percentage provided to other categories of employees with the same duration of training and almost equivalent diploma. Most of the nurses retire in the capacity in which they initially join. The Government of India had appointed a High Power Committee to look into the promotion, cadres, status and other grievances of the Nurses. A suggestions for expeditious cadre review has evoked no response. A system with inbuilt arrangement of allowing the next higher scale after every five years of service has been ignored by the government. Similarly, in case of engineers (Table 7) , it is noticed that the chances of promotion are higher (about 25 per cent) as against 10 per cent in case of the staff nurses. Secondly, the fraction of promotional opportunities for engineers are constant whereas the same for the nursing personnel decrease at an increasing rate. Thirdly, there is a glaring difference in pay scales of the nursing personnel and the engineers from the lowest to the highest rank. A Nursing Superintendent or a Principal Tutor is given the scale of Rs. 2200– 4000 but the Chief Engineer is allowed the scale of Rs. 4800–6300. Thus, the rare promotional prospects and the disparity in the pay scale kill the incentives of the nursing personnel. This is again responsible for the poor economic status of the nurses in society.

Besides wage structure and promotional opportunities, other incentives are special pay for specialised area, nursing allowance, messing allowance and non–practicing allowance etc. The Central Government have identified some areas where the nursing personnel working in particularly arduous or unpleasant jobs or hard specialised areas are eligible for special pay. But the same facilities have not been extended to nurses working with the State Government. Nursing allowance is not given. Messing allowance is paid in some States on the recommendation of the Third Pay Commission. Nursing Personnel are neither given non–practising allowance nor are they allowed to do private practice like doctors as is being done in the state like Orissa. It has been discussed before that the nursing personnel are required to perform more than 48 hours duty per week and that too without any overtime allowance. Apart from legal or moral considerations this goes against the natural justice. An overtime allowance could only compensate this loss. Similarly, they are not given official allowances for handling of the stores, managing accounts and keeping linen and other stocks of medicine as is being paid to cashiers. Night Duty allowance is being paid in P & T, Civil Aviation and Railways departments. But this allowance is not given to nurses on night duty all over the country. The system of washing and Uniform allowance, Railway concession, Transport facilities and conveyance allowances is not satisfactory in our State (Table 10).

Sources of Income

Service income, part–time income, private income and other sources of income constitute sources of income. All the sources of income are interdependent and interacting. Besides service income, part–time income is another source of income to enhance the socio–economic status of an individual. After toiling hard with a strainous routine a nurse would rarely show an inclination for taking up any part–time job like nursing in a clinic or the like. Economically

Table 10: Other Benefits provided to Nursing Personnel in Centre and various States

Sl. no.	*Benefits*	*Centre*	*Orissa*	*Karnataka*	*Andhra Pradesh*	*Maharashtra*	*Uttar Pradesh*	*Delhi*
1.	Uniform allowance	1500 p.a.	250 p.a.	30,40 & 50 p.m.	300 p.a.	360 p.a.	750 p.a.	150 p.m.
2.	Washing allowance	75 p.m.	–	–	15 p.m.	20 p.m.	20 p.m.	75 p.m.
3.	Nursing allowance	150 p.m.	–	–	–	–	–	50 pm.
4.	Messing allowance	–	–	–	–	90 p.m. –	–	
5.	Special pay at Operation Theatre	–	–	–	20 p.m.	30 p.m.	25 p.m.	–
6.	ICU special allowance	–	–	–	–	30 p.m.	–	60 p.m.
7.	Night super special pay for night sister	–	–	–	2 per day	30 p.m.	–	–
8.	Night duty staff nurse	–	–	–	–	–	–	–
9.	Mental hospital allowance	–	–	–	20 p.m.	20 p.m.	–	60 p.m.
10.	Special pay to Matrons	–	–	–	–	20 p.m.	–	–
11.	ESIS allowance	–	–	–	–	–	–	–
12.	Ration allowance	10%	–	75 p.m.	–	–	100 p.m.	–
13.	House Rent	–	10%	10%	10%	10%	250 p.m.	15 p.m.
14.	Stitching allowance	–	–	–	–	–	–	–
15.	NGGOS clinic allowance	–	–	–	–	25%	–	–
16.	Compensatory salary	–	–	15 days salary	–	–	–	–
17.	Time bound promotion	–	–	Once in service	Once in service	–	–	–
18.	Railway concession	–	–	–	–	–	–	–
19.	Crèche facilities	–	–	Available	–	–	–	Available

Source: Directorate of Health and Family Welfare, Government of Orissa.

speaking, the additional labour unit of nurses after the shift duty involves more and more marginal sacrifice which may not be compensated by any higher marginal earning. None of the nurses covered in this stage has any part–time income.

Almost all nurses have negative response towards private income. Firstly, private practice contravenes the service and conduct rules. On the other hand, they are unwilling to sacrifice their private time and energy to earn some extra income at home. After all, they have their children and the families and they do not like to jeopardise the family peace by taking up private assignments for a paltry sum of money which would in no way be a compensation for the sacrifice they make. It is found that most of the nurses are born and brought up in poor family. 92 per cent of the nurses belong to landless families and the rest 8 per cent have come from the families with marginal land base. A tight routine, lack of spare time and their femininity have further circumvented their scope for earning extra income.

Saving and Investment

Saving is necessary to meet unforeseen events in life, sickness and old age etc. Saving depends on two factors : willingness to save and ability to save. Ability to save depends upon the level of income and marginal propensity to consume. In other words, individual income determines his saving. One the other hand, investment depends upon the marginal efficiency of capital in relation to interest rate, the facilities of saving, the habit of the people, the political stability and the like. Ultimately all savings are mobilised in the form of investment.

While analysing the saving and investment pattern of the nurses, it is found from the Table 11, that only 357 (94.2) nurses have General Provident Fund (GPF), 11 (2.9) have Post Office savings and the rest have neither provident fund nor postal savings. This is because of the nature of appointment of their service (Fig. 5).

94.2 per cent of nurses, being the only earning members of the families have to support the dependants out of their meager income and have no capacity to save (Fig. 5). Marginal number of nurses (11 per cent) have their personal savings in the Post Offices and banks either in the form of savings deposits or in the form of

Table 11: Nurses according to Saving and Investment

medical college hospital	*G.P.F.*	*Postal Savings*	*Investments*
SCB	171 (96.1)	7 (3.9)	4 (2.2)
MKCG	93 (92.2)	2 (1.8)	Nil
VSS	93 (93.0)	2 (2.0)	Nil
Total	357 (94.2)	11 (2.9)	4 (0.9)

(Figures in the bracket indicate percentage of totals 379).

Cumulative Time Deposits. They are saving not because of domestic necessity, but because of their will to save. Saving and Investment of 2.2 per cent of nurses of SCB Medical College hospital is possible due to earnings of their husbands. Double income in the family necessarily increases their saving capacity to purchase equity in the companies. These are the exceptions because of the high income earner husbands who are either businessman or in very good jobs.

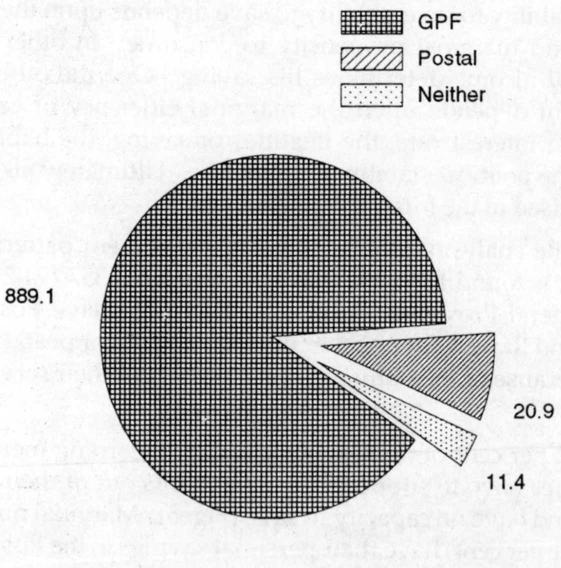

Fig. 5: Personal Savings of Nurses in three medical college hospitals.

Pattern of Expenditure

An analysis of the per capita income, assets and liabilities of the nurses would be of little use in our study. Hence an attempt is made here to study the pattern of expenditures to evaluate their economic status in society. The different parameters used to evaluate the pattern of expenditures are (1) trade expenses, (2) conveyance expenses, (3) family expenses, (4) expenses for children, (5) medical expenses and (6) miscellaneous expenses.

Nurses have to incur some trade expenses peculiar to their profession alone. For instance, they have to incur some regular expenses for the proper maintenance of their immaculately white dress and the apron. Those in the infectious wards spend something to protect themselves from some possible attack by viruses and germs. Besides, they also keep a small portion of their budget for tea, coffee and the like during the tidious duty hours to break the monotony and provide themselves some relief from the strains of the nerves. The range of trade expenses in the three medical college hospitals varies from 10 per cent to 17 per cent. On an average it is 10 per cent, 13.8 per cent and 14.2 per cent in SCB, MKCG and VSS Medical College hospital respectively. Differences in expenses or responses are primarily due to the difference in costs of the food articles. Conveyance expenses are very common to all employees. The mode of conveyance determines the expenditure under this head.

53.6 per cent of the sample nurses are provided with accommodation in the hospital campuses and the rest 46.4 per cent bear the burden of conveyance in the absence of any provision of conveyance allowance to the State Government employees. In SCB Medical College hospital 88 (49.4 per cent) nurses come from outside ranging from a distance of one km to 40 kms though one is expected to remain within the permitted limit of eight kms from the campus. This they do either because of availability of cheap accommodation or because of family ties. Some nurses reside at Bhubaneswar and Choudwar which are for all practical purposes treated as suburbs of the city of Cuttack. In the case of VSS hospital 45 (44.6 per cent) nurses reside outside the hospital campus and incur heavy expenses because of the distance and the unsatisfactory mode of transport. On an average 16.2 per cent of their total expenses are incurred on this head. This expenditure is relatively low per cent (9.2) in case of nurses of MKCG hospital. In case of SCB Medical College hospital it is still lower per cent (8.0) because of the cheap mode of conveyance.

The average monthly expenditure are classified under five groups such as food, clothing, fuel and lighting, ceremonies and miscellaneous expenses. It is against their wish they spend less on baby care and baby food. Even when there is no necessity of baby food because of the absence of small kids and there is the necessity of incurring expenditure on the education of the grown up children, they are not able to meet it due to their budget constraints. They hardly spend 4–5 per cent of their income on the educational expenses of their children. Their medical expenses are not much because they belong to the medical team. It is 2.5 per cent on the average. They might be incurring same expenditure to meet unforeseen events.

Rest of the expenses include purchase of assets, bonds and meeting expenses in ceremonial occasions. It is greater in case of nurses of SCB Medical College hospital because of regular guests in Cuttack city. It is minor component of total expenses. Economically speaking only the lower income people spend major portion of their income in food consumption as their marginal propensity to consume is high. The study reveals the fact that nurses in all medical college hospitals spend their lion share in food and family expenses. Some have reservations to enumerate their expectations about their pay scales and other allowances in relation to load of work and others want an enhancement in their pay and perks to counter the inflationary pressures. Pensions are calculated on the basic pay which is very low and allowances are not taken into account for that purpose. The nurses approaching their age of superannuation view the moment with a sigh of despair. Upto 1966, they were given a very low scale of pay which is slightly improved with the revision of pay in 1976 and 1985. A proposal was made again to revise their scale of pay to bring it at par with that of the centre with effect from Ist January, 1989 retrospectively and it has been given effect to. After revision of pay scale, their economic condition is slightly better up. But there is also same disparities in their scale and economic status has no improvement.

3.3 Organisation and Composition of Nurses

Nurse is the most crucial component of the health care team. One of the major problems facing the health and nursing administrators in India today is the problem of providing qualitative nursing personnel in adequate number. As on 31st December, 1989, there were 2,07,430 registered nurses and 1,08,511 auxiliary nurse midwives (ANM) in India against the projected need of 9,59,980 nurses by the year 2000. The pay scale, status and general working conditions of the nurses require considerable improvement to attract superior talents to this service in adequate number.

The Director General of Health Services at the Centre directly controls the nursing personnel and their services. The Nursing Advisor assisted by a Nursing Officer and a supporting staff is held directly accountable to the Deputy Director General (DDG). She advises the Government on all matters relating to nursing services and nursing education etc. The present position of the Nursing Advisor in the organisational set up of the Directorate General of Health Services is presented in Fig. 6.

The Directorates of Health Services in the States look after the nursing services and nursing education. In most of the States nurses look after only the hospital nursing services and schools of nursing attached to the hospitals. The community nursing components including training of auxiliary midwives are looked after by a doctor in the Maternal and Child Welfare Division. In West Bengal, Gujarat, Karnataka, Kerala, Maharashtra and Orissa one and some times more than one nurses are posted at the Directorate level. The post of District Public Health Nurse has been created under the family welfare programme. She is expected to look after all health visitors and ANM working in her district in Primary Health Centres.

Organisation of Nursing Services in Orissa

It is interesting to trace the historical background of State Nursing Services in Orissa. Initially nursing services were not controlled by the Government but were controlled by independent bodies administered by prominent public personalities and philanthropists and consequently, the government had no financial stake in it. The prime function of these private bodies in fact, was

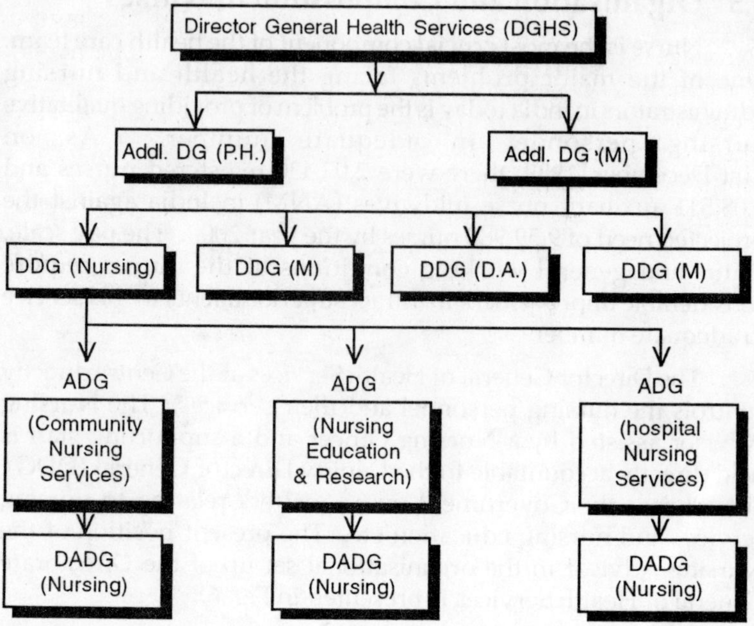

Fig. 6: Nursing Organisational set up at National Level.

to provide nursing services to the Government hospitals and run the nursing education programme. The financial liabilities of the organisation was being borne by Christian missionaries and the agents called **"non–sisters"**.

During this period nursing services were rendered by religious nurse of the **"All Saint Order"**. The first supervisor sister to work in a hospital was sister **"Barbara"**. At that time trained nurses in Orissa had to work on a contract basis. But gradually with the increase in the financial burden nursing services became disorganised after independence. In the year 1961 the State Government brought the nursing services to its fold and so was born the services in Orissa. Thereafter, the Orissa Nursing Council and Nursing Examination Board were established.

Orissa, at present has a full–fledged State Nursing Organisation having different local branches. There are three college hospitals in Orissa, located at Cuttack, Berhampur and Sambalpur having Chief Matron as the nursing executive head.

Besides these three college hospitals, three Government Nursing Schools are also functioning in SCB Medical College, Cuttack, VSS Medical College, Burla and MKCG Medical College, Berhampur. A college of nursing has also been established recently at Berhampur for conducting B.Sc. Nursing Course. But there is no facility of Post–Graduate teaching in the State. In the pre–independence days, the position of the Nursing Staff was still more unsatisfactory. The number of nurses employed in public medical institutions in the different provinces is given in Table 12.

Table 12: Number of Nurses Employed before Independence (1943)

Province	*Medical Institutions*					
	Rural			*Urban*		
	European and Anglo–Indian	*Indian*	*Total*	*European and Anglo–Indian*	*Indian*	*Total*
Bengal	13	29	42	392	536	928
Bihar	17	26	43	97	196	293
Bombay	2	42	44	211	957	1168
Central Provinces and Beral	4	25	29	31	177	208
Madras and North West Frontier	1	12	13	5	94	99
Orissa	3	4	7	11	27	38
Sind	–	–	103	–	–	–
United Provinces	–	–	257	–	–	–
Assam	–	48	48	14	–	14
Delhi	–	–	–	104	200	304

Source: Indian Nursing Year Book (INYB), 1982.

The position reflects an unsatisfactory State of affairs so much so that it would be inconceivable in the European Countries and in the USA where proper nursing is always regarded as an essential part of modern medical practice. In 1943, the optimum ratio of nurses to hospital beds in these countries was 2.5 : 1. Compared to this, the total number of nurses employed in some provinces in India was hardly sufficient to provide adequate nursing staff for even a single five hundred bedded hospital of Orissa and Sind. After nearly half a century Orissa has not made any significant progress in this regard in comparison to States like Maharashtra and Kerala. The present number and pay scales of nurses in Orissa is presented in Table 13.

Table 13: Nursing Personnel according to Designation (1988–89)

Designation	*No. of post*	*Vacancy*	*Scale of pay*
Staff Nurse	1563	Nil	1350 — 2200
Nursing Sister/ O.T. Nurse/ Psychiatric Nurse	153	8	1400 — 2300
Assistant Matron/ Public Health Nurse/ Sister Nurse	22	4	1600 — 2600
Matron	3	2	2000 — 3500
Chief Matron (Gazetted Class–II)	3	3	2200 — 4000
Staff Nurse* (Selection Grade)	–	–	1400 — 2300

* Those who are experienced but no promotion due to non–availability of vacancy will be regarded as Selection Grade Staff Nurse.

Source: Directorate of Health Services, Government of Orissa.

The Table reveals that there are 1,744 posts in the Orissa Nursing Organisation out of which 17 posts are lying vacant at present. The Chief Matrons of three medical college hospitals are in the rank of Class II State service. The Organisational set up at the Directorate level is given in the Fig 7. Fig. 8 depicts the hierarchic set up of organisation in school and colleges. Principal Tutors in the Nursing Schools are Class II Officers but in Berhampur Nursing college, the Principal is a Class I Officer and its Lecturers are Class II Officers of state Government.

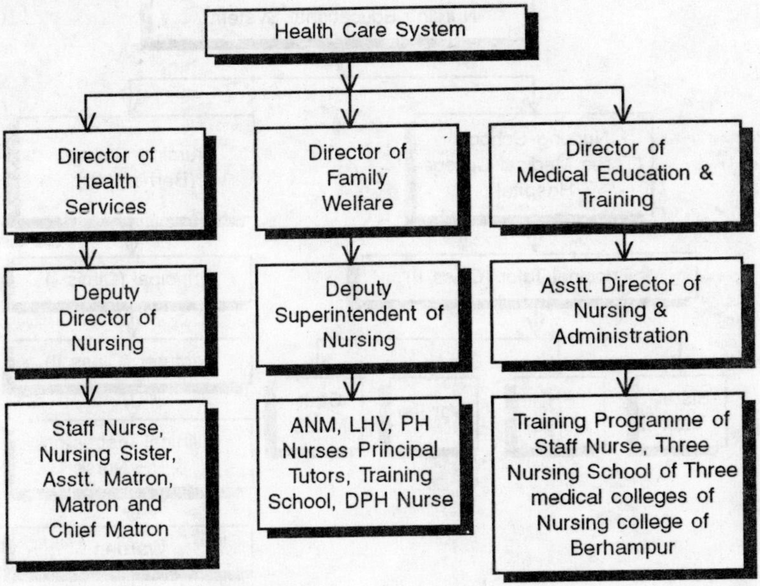

Fig. 7: Organisational set up in Orissa

Composition of Nursing Personnel in the three Medical College Hospitals

This section gives a general picture of the nursing personnel, *i.e.*, their number, their distribution according to age, sex, religion, marital status, domicile and experience etc. of the three medical college hospitals of Orissa. Table 14 gives the distribution of the existing staff employed in the three medical college hospitals of Orissa according to the their status. The table also reveals that the post of Chief Matron is lying vacant in all the three college hospitals. There is only one Matron in SCB Medical College hospital and the other two posts in the other two college hospitals are lying vacant. However, there is one Assistant Matron in each of the three medical college hospitals.

Table 14 reveals that under each Assistant Matron in the three medical college hospitals the number of nursing sisters working is 31, 18 and 17 respectively and the number of staff nurse working is 145, 82 and 82 respectively. The number of nurses in three medical college hospitals and other Government hospitals and dispensaries are represented in Fig 9.

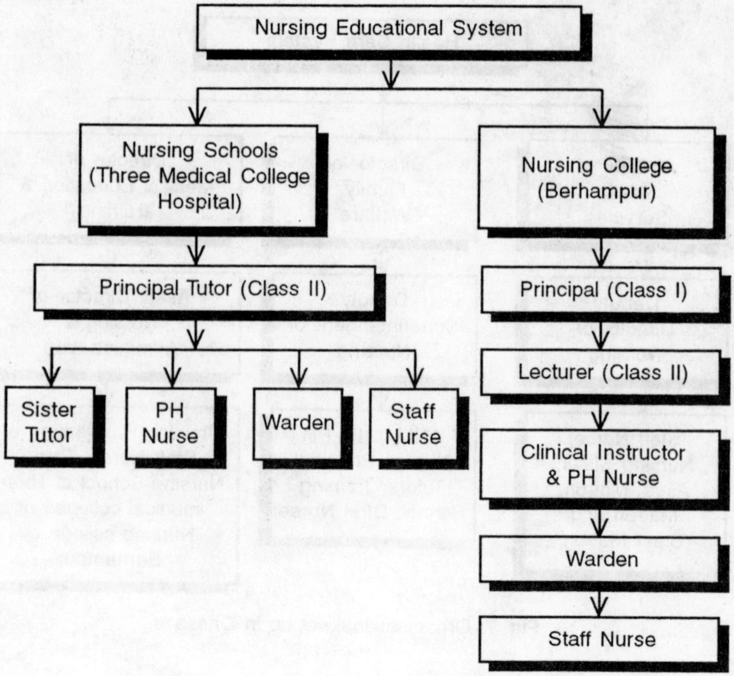

Fig. 8: Organisational set up in Nursing Schools

Table 14: Status of Nursing Population

Designation	*Medical College Hospitals*			*Total*	*Percentage to total*
	SCB	*MKCG*	*VSS*		
Chief Matron	–	–	–	–	–
Matron	1	–	–	1	0.02
Asst. Matron	1	1	1	3	0.8
Nursing Sister	31	18	17	66	17.5
Staff Nurse	145	82	82	309	81.5
Total	178 (10.2)	101 (5.8)	100 (5.7)	379 (21.7)	100

(1) Figures in the bracket indicate percentage to the total nursing personnel (1,744) in the State.

(2) Figures in the last column indicate percentage to the total (379) nurses in college hospitals of Orissa.

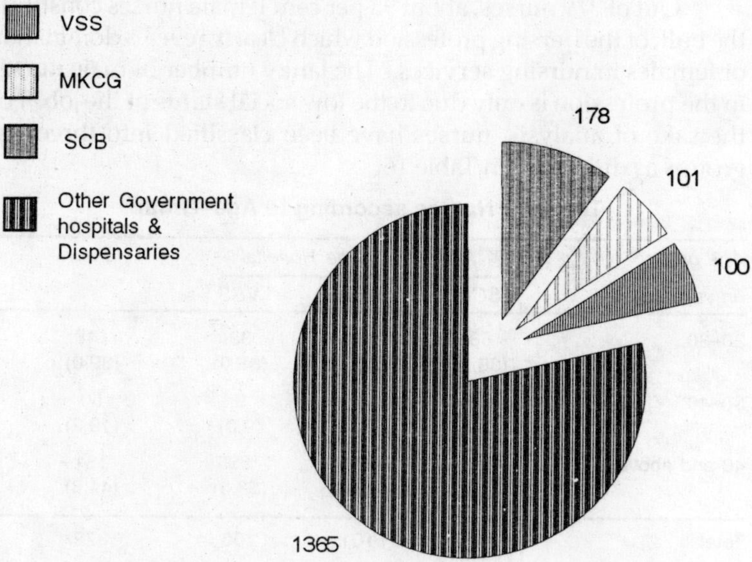

Fig. 9: Number of nurses in three medical college hospitals of Orissa.

Sex Ratio, Age–Group and Marital Status

The profession from the beginning was run by females who are by nature and temperament eminently suited for the kind of services required in this field. There is the lone case of a physically handicapped male staff nurse in SCB Medical College hospital and their number is only four and three in MKCG medical hospital and VSS Medical College hospital respectively. The position is given in Table 15.

Table 15: Nurses according to Sex

Sex	*Medical College Hospitals*			*Total*
	SCB	*MKCG*	*VSS*	
Female	177	97	97	371 (97.9)
Male	1	4	3	8 (2.1)
Total	178	101	100	379

(Figures in the bracket in total column indicate percentage to the total 379).

Out of 379 nurses, about 98 per cent female nurses constitute the bulk of the nursing profession which clearly reveals domination of females in nursing services. The lanky number of male nurses in the profession is only due to the low social status of the job. For the sake of analysis, nurses have been classified into three age groups as discussed in Table 16.

Table 16: Nurses according to Age–Group

Age group (in years)	*Medical College Hospital*			*Total*
	SCB	*MKCG*	*VSS*	
20–30	68 (38.2)	47 (46.5)	33 (33.0)	148 (39.0)
30–40	26 (14.6)	15 (14.9)	9 (9.0)	50 (19.2)
40 and above	84 (47.2)	39 (38.6)	58 (58.0)	181 (41.8)
Total	178	101	100	379

(Figures in the bracket indicate percentage to total 379.

Table 16 reveals that 39 per cent of nurses belong to the age group of 20–30. Almost all nurses of this age group are young diploma holders completing a three and half year general nursing and midwifery course. Only 19 per cent of nurses are in the age group of 30 to 40. This is only because of the suspension of regular appointment during the period 1965–1978. More than 41 per cent of nurses belong to the third category (40 and above). Massive expansion of nursing services by the Christian Missionaries is responsible for large number of nurses in this age group today. Nurses of the age group of 20–30 and 30–40 are staff nurses. Some of them also have completed 20 years of their services as staff nurses. Their number constitute bulk of the profession, say, about 40 per cent. Such a large number of nurses are stagnating because of lack of promotional avenues. All specialised nurses like psychiatric and O.T. nurses fall in the age group of 40 and above. The age group structure of nurses in three medical college hospitals is represented in Fig 10.

Marital status is an important parameter of social status of nurses. There is a growing trend of late marriage among the nursing community. Table 17 reveals the composition of nurses according to their marital status.

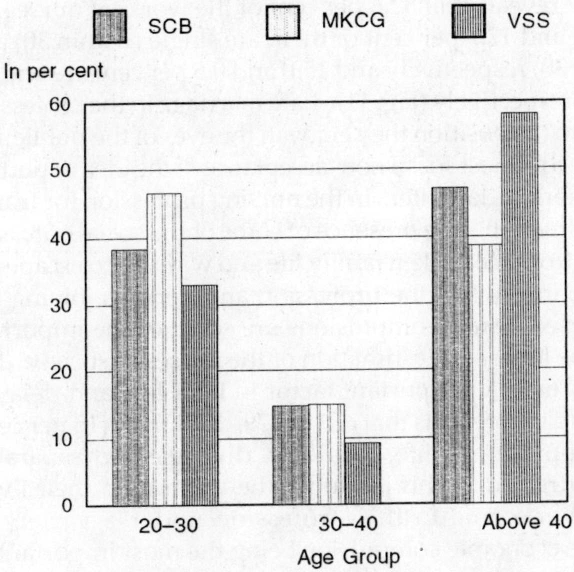

Fig. 10: Age Composition of Nurses.

Table 17: Composition of Nurses according to their Marital Status

Marital Status	*Medical College Hospitals*			*Total*
	SCB	*MKCG*	*VSS*	
Married	85 (47.8)	62 (61.1)	52 (52.0)	199 (52.6)
Single (within 30)	26 (14.6)	12 (11.9)	16 (16.0)	54 (14.2)
Single (after 30)	34 (19.1)	17 (16 8)	16 (16.0)	67 (17.7)
Widow	33 (18.5)	10 (9.9)	4 (4.0)	57 (15.0)
Divorced	Nil	Nil	2 (2.0)	2 (0.5)
Total	178	101	100	379

(Figures in the bracket indicate percentage to the total of the respective institution and figures in bracket in Total column indicate percentage to the total of all the three institutions).

Table 17 reveals that 52.6 per cent of the working nurses are married, 14.2 and 17.7 per cent of them are single (within 30) and single (above 30) respectively and 15.0 and 0.5 per cent are widow and divorcee respectively (Fig. 11). Late marriage in the profession is partly due to the position they enjoy in the eyes of the public and the partly due to almost social non–acceptance of the idea of putting the wives, sisters or daughters in the nursing profession for fear of low social estimation. The presence of some of the social outcastes the run away from the broken family life and widows to escape the torture of the in–laws in the profession and persons joining the service under economic compulsions are some of the important reasons for the low social estimation of the nurses in society. The low social status is an important factor in their late and delayed marriages. Table 17 reveals that out of 379, 57 nurses (15 per cent) had an unhappy family life. Widows, divorcee and separated women are attracted to this job to fill the vacuum in their lives. Many, however, come to this profession under a variety of situations, the economic compulsion being the most important of them.

Religion, Language and Domicile

Hindus are in majority in the profession. Muslims and Christians have their share in very small proportions (Fig. 12). There was a popular belief in the past that only Christians come to the nursing profession. Some of the research findings also support this view and it is observed that Christian women were more attracted to the nursing profession than those of any other community. Persons belonging to Buddhist and other religious faith are conspicuous by their absence in the present population (Table 18).

It may be observed from the above Table that 82.3 per cent of the population are Hindus and 17.7 per cent belong to the Christian community. There is not a single nurse belonging to Muslim or any other religion. Religious composition of nurses is represented in Fig 12. It clearly reveals the intra religious disparities between three hospitals. But the disparities are marginal because of homogeneous service conditions. Of the 379 nurses, 361 are Oriya, four are Bengali, six are Telugu and eight are Keralies. This indicates the dominance of local girls in the profession in all the three medical college hospitals of Orissa. All non–Oriya nurses, because of their

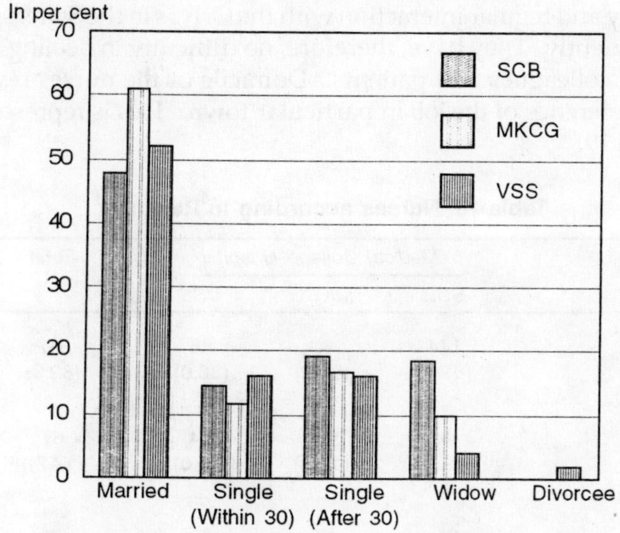

Fig. 11: Nurses by Marital Status.

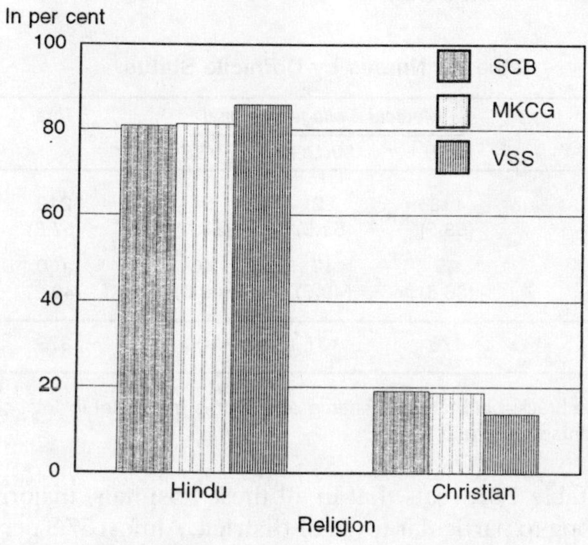

Fig. 12: Religious Composition of Nurses.

long stay and regular interaction with the Oriyas in the State, speak Oriya fluently. They have, therefore, no difficulty in dealing with friends, colleagues and patients. Domicile of the nurses reveals their preference of the job in particular town. This is represented in Table 19.

Table 18: Nurses according to Religion

Religion	*Medical College Hospital*			*Total*
	SCB	*MKCG*	*VSS*	
Hindu	144 (81.0)	82 (81.2)	86 (86.0)	312 (82.3)
Muslim	–	–	–	–
Christian	34 (19.0)	19 (18.8)	14 (14.0)	67 (17.7))
Buddhists	–	–	–	–
Others	–	–	–	–
Total	178	101	100	379

(Figures in the bracket indicate percentage and figures in bracket in total column indicate percentage to grand total).

Table 19: Nurses by Domicile Status

Domicile	*Medical College Hospital*			*Total*
	SCB	*MKCG*	*VSS*	
Local	113 (63.5)	52 (51.5)	54 (54.0)	219 (57.8)
Outsiders	65 (36.5)	49 (48.5)	46 (46.0)	160 (42.2)
Total	178	101	100	379

(Figures in the bracket indicate percentage and figures in bracket in Total column indicate percentage to grand total).

The Table 19 reveals that in all these hospitals, majority of nurses belong to particular town or district. Almost 57.8 per cent of nurses belong to their respective towns or their periphery. From among them some are born and brought up in that particular area and others have migrated in search of better employment opportunities and have become the residents of those particular localities.

Education and Work Experience

A nurse is appointed as a staff nurse after qualifying in General Nursing and Midwifery Course as per rules. All the sample nurses, therefore, have completed three and half years of General Nursing and Midwifery course. Of course, norms and conditions have been partially modified now. Table 20 indicates the educational status of existing nurses in the hospitals.

Table 20: Nurses by Educational Status

Educational Status	*Medical College Hospital*			*Total*
	SCB	*MKCG*	*VSS*	
M.E.	104 (38.4)	61 (60.4)	67 (67.0)	232 (61.2)
H.S.C.	71 (39.9)	37 (36.6)	31 (31.0)	139 (36.7)
+2 Sc. or +2 Arts	2 (1.1)	3 (2.9)	2 (2.0)	7 (1.8)
B.A.	1 (0.6)	–	–	1 (0.3)
Total	178	101	100	379

(Figures in the bracket indicate percentage and figures in bracket in Total column indicate percentage to grand total).

Table 20 reveals that of the 379 nurses 232 (61.2 per cent) have education upto M.E. standard constituting the bulk of the nursing profession. On the contrary only one (0.3 per cent) of the nurses is a graduate. Nearly one third of the nursing profession (36.7 per cent) have gone upto H.S.C. standard. This disparity is in the educational qualification is only due to change of norms and conditions of the Government of Orissa from time to time (1961–86) (Fig. 13). But there is no such alarming differences in between college hospitals as regards to qualification.

Form the study of occupational history of the nurses, it is noticed that 373 nurses were not employed elsewhere prior to their

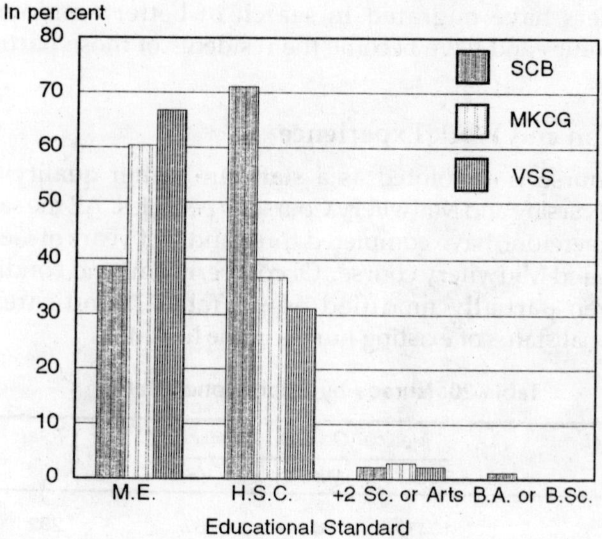

Fig. 13: Educational Status of Nurses.

joining in the present jobs. On the whole occupational mobility is negligible. They think that the special training they receive and the skill they acquire could be better and properly utilised only if they continue as such and go on rendering their services to the society. Only six nurses had previously worked in private hospitals and entered into the government hospital later. Work experience of nurses is an indicator of the quality of services they render. Viewed from this angle, all Sister Tutors, Nursing Sister and Matrons have more than 20 years of experience. Because of their fairly long experience their views and observations are always given due weightage. Their composition is revealed in Table 21.

About 32.2 per cent nurses have less than 10 years of experience. Similarly, 33 per cent of nurses have experience between 10 and 20 years and 34.8 per cent have more than 20 years of experience. Experienced nurses have given a variety of reasons for their acceptance of the job. Some of them feel the urge of serving the society in this way and claim to be derived a sort of psychological satisfaction by sharing the joys and sorrows of the patients. Some others have accepted it for the maximum utilisation of their special

Table 21: Nurses according to Years of Experience

Years of Experience	*Medical College Hospital*			*Total*
	SCB	*MKCG*	*VSS*	
0–10	53 (29.8)	35 (34.7)	34 (34.0)	122 (32.2)
10–20	61 (31.3)	34 (33.7)	30 (30.0)	125 (33.0)
20 and above	64 (36.0)	32 (31.7)	36 (36.0)	132 (34.8)
Total	178	101	100	379

(Figures in the bracket indicate percentage and figures in bracket in Total column indicate percentage to grand total).

training and education for the benefit of the nation. Special fascination for the job might have attracted a section of nurses to this noble profession. The parameters like marital status, domicile status, educational status, family set up and work experiences are certain indices of social status. All these are interacting with one another to measure the social status of nurses. Besides that, organisational structure of the State is in obscurity. It may be concluded from the structure that though nursing is a profession of paramount importance within the national health delivery system, yet it has been deliberately deprived of the due status for some extraneous considerations.

Chapter 4
Working and Living Conditions

The ever growing demand of trained nurses is the natural outcome of the efforts made to meet the present day challenges in this front. A balance needs be struck between the demand for and supply of nurses in society in order to ensure a socio–economic equilibrium. New blood are to be inducted into the profession and there must be sufficient incentive for the old to continue so as to give the cadre the necessary number and strength to cater to the expanding social needs. Attainment of this objective presupposes agreeable working and living conditions.

Variables like job satisfaction, employees' attitude and morale have acquired an important place in the literature of industrial, vocational and social psychology. The terms **"job satisfaction"**, **"job attitudes"** and **"morale"** are used inter–changeably for effective orientations of individuals towards their present work roles. Likerts and Willits define job morale as "an individual's mental attitude towards all features of his work and towards all the people with whom he works". Similarly, Guion defines morale as "the extent to which the individual perceives that satisfaction as stemming from his total job situation".

Society is assured of a regular supply of excellent nursing service and improved health standard provided the nurse has a high morale or a positive attitude and conditions are conducive for her to derive job satisfaction. Government as an ideal employer expect the nursing personnel to be loyal, punctual and hard working. It even expects certain degree of dedication and sacrifice from them. The nurses and the employer are aware of each others expectations. But there is direction relationship between working conditions offered to employees and their job satisfaction. Nurses may work effectively provided the employer provides ideal working conditions which include clean, hygienic and decent work place with all the necessary facilities; suitable and reasonable working hours; a decent salary and allowances; a set of acceptable rules on transfer, promotion and leave; accommodation transportation, telephone and welfare facilities like medical facilities and maternity benefit; appreciation of efficient services; an air of democracy in the organisation; freedom of association and encouragement for workers' participation in management; absence of discrimination on any ground and a guarantee on the right of collective bargaining. Excellent working conditions may help in reducing the number of disputes between the workers and the management and encourage smooth conduct of work.

According to Vroom, the major determinants of job satisfaction are as follows:

(i) Hours of work,

(ii) Supervision,

(iii) The work group,

(iv) Job Content,

(v) Wages and

(vi) Promotional opportunities.

In addition to these direct factors, other important factors influencing the worker's attitude towards the job are stated below:

(i) Job Security,

(ii) Opportunity to work and make collective bargaining.

(iii) Guidance from superiors,

(iv) Communication,

(v) Delegation of authority,

(vi) Physical facilities at work place,

(vii) Occupational health protection,

(viii) Welfare facilities and

(ix) Balanced Organisational set up.

These determinants of job satisfaction are different conditions of employment to work. Every employer ought to have mastered the skill of managing effectively these determinants to keep the employees contented and peaceful. Nurses working in the medical college hospitals are part of the medical organisation in Orissa. "An organisation is a social system where people join together in some sort of formal structure to achieve an objective, and an organisation develops". Generally, people use some sort of formal technology to achieve their objective. There is, therefore, an interaction of people's technology and structure in the organisation. All these three elements are influenced by the external social system and they in turn influence it. The people–the living, thinking, feelings beings–who create the organisation constitute the internal social system of the organisation. Similarly, there is an interaction between the nurses, the formal structure and their formal technology to achieve the objective (Fig. 14).

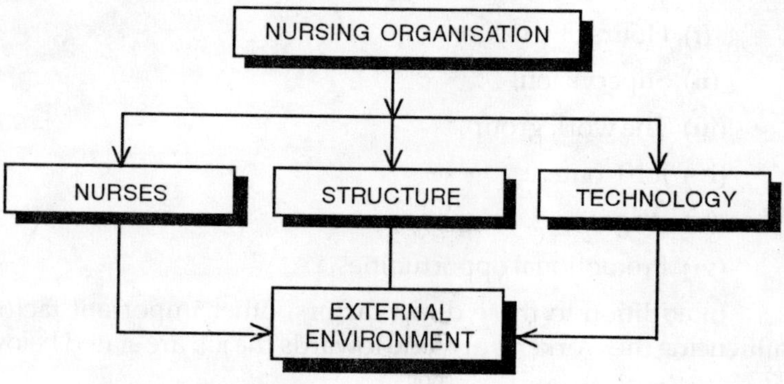

Fig. 14: Key Elements in Organisational Behaviour.

The diagram depicts the key elements of nursing organisation. Nurses, structure and technology (three elements) are represented as three peak points. They are interacting with one another and collectively influence external environment.

From the figure it is also noticed that all nurses in the organisation are interested in improving the human behaviour in the organisation as it relates to structure, technology and the external social system but the management has more responsibility in this respect. It has to develop an environment in which nurses are motivated to team work that effectively fulfils their own needs and also achieves organisational objectives. The task of management is not to push or drive employees due to release inner drives that nurses already have. In an organisation, the management has to motivate employees by treating them differently according to their need, situation and environment. Every employee has certain physiological or primary needs and some social or psychological needs called the secondary needs. The physiological needs like food, water, sleep, air to breathe and satisfactory temperature arising out of basic physiology of life are important for survival and they are universal among the people. Secondary needs are higher order needs of the mind and spirit rather than of physical body such as rivalry, self–esteem, sense of duty and belongingness etc. These needs vary among people much more than primary needs. Secondary needs are often hidden so that a person cannot recognise them and he attributes his dissatisfaction to something more tangible, such as wages. Needs have certain levels of priority. These are as mentioned below.

(i) Basic physiological needs,

(ii) Safety and Security,

(iii) Belonging and Social needs,

(iv) Esteem and Status, and

(v) Self actualisation and fulfilment.

Order of priority of human needs may be represented in figure (Fig. 15). Need level has a definite sequence of domination. For example, unless basic physiological needs are reasonably satisfied, need number 2 does not dominate. In the early USA history physiological needs, safety and security were dominant but now they are fairly satisfied and higher level needs tend to dominate there. This trend suggests that satisfaction of primary needs does not produce contentment, instead it unleashes a new series of discontents. The secondary needs now begin to acquire the power to motivate. People do not stop wanting, but when they have food, water and air, they want in succession, safety, love, esteem and self–fulfilment (Fig. 16). It is well known that in real situation all needs interact together within a whole person. They also tend to develop and combine. It might be useful to assume a typical

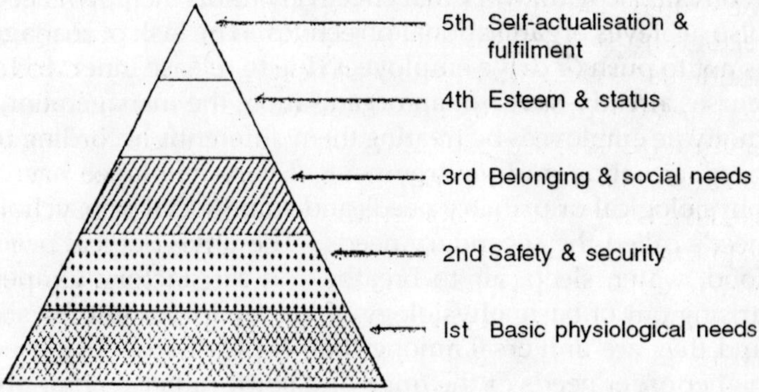

Fig. 15: Order of priority of human needs according to Maslow.

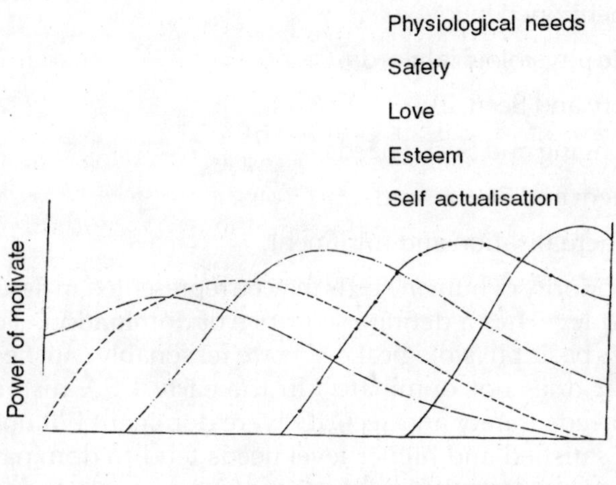

Fig. 16: Psychological development.

situation of the Indian worker proposed by Maslow with the five need level interacting within him.

There is a direction relationship between the satisfaction of wants or needs and the job satisfaction of the employee. Job behaviour and the quality of the work done depends on job satisfaction. According to Vroom, "the more satisfied a worker, the stronger the force on him to remain in his job. There is negative relationship between job satisfaction and resignations, absences and accidents". Therefore, a steady, efficient, excellent and reductive performance from an employee can be expected by creation of an environment in the organisation which would help each employee to satisfy his different types of needs. It may be observed that satisfaction of basic physiological needs is directly related to wages or physical facilities at the work place. Second order needs of safety and security are related to job security and occupational health protection. Similarly, satisfaction of the remaining different types of needs depend on some aspect or the other of the working conditions of the employee which is one of the determinants of their job satisfaction. The employer must be able to handle these determinants of job satisfaction successfully.

Another useful way to think about money as a reward might be envisioned from the expectancy model. Expectancy theory States that Valence x Expectancy = Motivation. Thus, if money is to act as a motivatior, an employee must want more of it (**Valence**) and also believe that the reward will follow by better performance (**Expectancy**). It might be safe to say that money is important to the typical Indian employee for a number of reasons. Money is needed to satisfy the lower level needs and is also a medium of social change. Moreover, it is a status value when it is received and spent. It is also an indicator of the employee's relative status.

The person brings to a situation only one blade and the other blade is what the situation brings to the person. It is only as the blades come together that the pattern behaviour is cut. Different situations are revealed round the world lead to varied job functions and employee's expectations. Within these situations, there are a multitude of variables in a complex relationship. Possible interactions among them are as limitless as the stars in the universe. Like all other individuals, we grow in a culture with its own typical socio–economic dimensions, human beliefs, customs, knowledge and practices (Fig.17). We accept the conventional socio–economic behaviour of our society and it influences all our actions even though it seldom enters into our conscious thinking.

The present study reflects various aspects of nurses' work role and working conditions in the medical college hospitals of

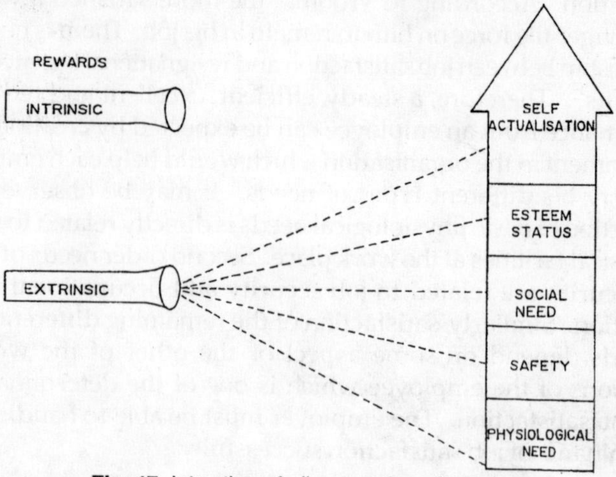

Fig. 17: Intraction of all categories of needs.

Orissa as well as living conditions of nurses in Orissa. Quality of work depends upon several factors like Working hours, Holidays and Leave, Supervision, Decision making, Work group, Level and status of employee, Specialisation, Promotional opportunities, Wages, Transfer, Job security, Nurses' Union, Delegation of authority, Physical facilities at work place, Occupational health protection and Welfare facilities.

4.1 Working Hours and Work Group

Nurses normally work for more than eight hours. There are nurses who work for more than ten hours. The Indian Nursing Council Act (INCA), 1957 provides that a nurse has to work for eight hours per day, but actually they work for longer hours. It implies that they are grossly over–worked and may have to suffer from its bad effects like too much tension and fatigue, lack of congenial atmosphere in the wards, deterioration in the quality of medical care of the patients and reduction in job satisfaction. They have to keep on standing near the sickbeds in an environment of germs, diseases and death and that makes some of them susceptible to nervous debility. Considering from the angle of physical and mental strains and long hours of work, the nurses can be said to have rendering a much useful service to society in comparison to that of other employees in other occupations.

The work schedule of nurses is completely specific unlike the normal office schedule. In all the three medical college hospitals there are shift duties for the nurses, the timing being 7.30 am to 3 pm, 3 pm to 9.30 pm and 9 pm to 7.30 am (next morning). The nature of the profession being something special dealing with life and death at every moment, a nurse cannot accept her work schedule to be as simple, specific and convenient as the normal office schedule. It is really tedious for the married nurses and those having small children to report to duty early in the morning and then again at night. Duties or shifts change by the office according to the needs of the hospital and load of work; but notice of the change in duty schedule is not given to them sufficiently in advance. Yet all of them adjust with it as a normal routine of their service life. Thus, abnormal work schedule with abnormal work load sometime make the situation not very palatable for the nursing personnel.

Shortage of nursing personnel is one of the important causes of the extra load of work. According to INCA, there should be one nurse for eight hours for five patients in a non–teaching institution. The prescribed ideal is one nurse for three beds for a teaching institution. But medical college hospital reports reveal that there is one nurse for thirty beds. Compared with the requirements of medical and health care facilities in the medical college hospitals, the number of nurses appears to be quite small. While the number of sanctioned posts remain almost constant for every hospital, there is an ever increasing flow of patients into it. With the wards already packed to their capacity, the hospitals can–not refuse admission to serious patients. A visit to these hospitals makes one aware of the stark reality. Every available floor space in the wards is occupied by the patients. Official records also bear a clear testimony to the astounding number of patients admitted and treated in each ward. The figure is many times more than the sanctioned beds in the wards. But the appointment of more number of nurses is not so easy as the admission of patients. Consequently, the existing staff have to serve unspecified number of patients admitted into the hospitals. The INCA, 1935 is totally ignored due to extra load of patients. The three medical college hospitals under study situated in the three revenue and geographical zones of the state with specified services are regularly attracting an increasing flow of serious patients. It can be easily marked from the table (Table 22) representing the state–wise nurse–patient ratio.

Table 22: State–wise Nurse–patient Ratio

Sates	*1 : 2*	*1 : 3*	*1 : 5*	*1 : 6*	*1 : 8*	*1 : 10*	*1 : more*	*Total response*
Andhra Pradesh	6	32	–	–	–	10	356	404
Bihar	–	12	–	–	–	37	–	49
Chandigarh	–	–	23	–	–	16	–	39
Delhi	8	3	1	–	–	5	–	17
Goa	2	–	2	1	5	–	75	85
Gujarat	84	138	40	–	–	50	91	331
Haryana	24	–	10	–	–	37	9	80
Himachal Pradesh	–	–	–	–	–	–	2	2
Kerala	16	–	–	8	–	–	–	24
Madras	–	–	–	–	–	–	5	5
Maharashtra	476	99	120	–	–	84	23	802
Orissa	**2**	**1**	–	–	–	**1**	**36**	**40**
Punjab	3	23	49	–	–	68	100	243
Total	621	308	245	9	5	308	625	2,121

Source: Trained Nurses' Association of India (TNAI) Survey Report, 1980.

Table 22 clearly reveals the Nurse–patient ratio of different states. In Orissa 36 nurses (90 per cent) have to work for more than 10 beds. But such a situation or ratio is completely absent in Bihar, Chandigarh, Delhi, Himachal Pradesh and Kerala. Only three (7.5 per cent) nurses have a situation of ILO standard in a sample survey of 40 nurses by TNAI. Extra load of clerical work like keeping various records of the patients, checking and keeping registers of medicines, stock of equipments, linen, utensil, food etc. imposes some additional burden (hours of work) on them. Such types of work have not only become a part and parcel of their duty; but it also takes away a good deal of their time and energy to non–nursing services. Consumers favour an immediate scrapping of the non–nursing work for the benefit of the patients and society as well.

Besides working hours in the hospitals, they spend sometime in travelling to the place of work and back home. About 50 per cent of the nurses are accommodated within the college hospital campus and the rest are seeking private accommodation who normally depend on cycle rickshaw or the public transport system to travel to their work place. In case of nurses of VSS Medical College, because it is economical, most of them prefer to travel by own bus even though it is inconvenient in some respects. A balance is struck between the cost of travelling and the time required to reach the hospital. Most of the nurses who come from lower middle class families cannot afford for better conveyance like taxi or having their own vehicle every day and consequently have to spend more time in travlling to their work place and back.

Overtime is a common phenomenon among nurses just like industrial workers. But the difference lies with the legal sanction and payment of workers. All the nurses of the three hospitals unanimously dealt on the difficulty and the impossibility of keeping the record of overtime work because it is a day–to–day problem and has almost become a routine for them. Neither they themselves nor the hospital management bother to keep any record of that. Consequently, no overtime payment is made to them either in cash or in kind and n o step has ever been taken to compensate them for the extra hours of work they are doing so ungrudgingly without demanding a monetary reward in return. Night duty is one of the peculiarities of the nursing profession. They have to do night duty for twelve hours with its concomitant physical and mental strain and serve the stick at these odd hours as a part of their routine. No financial compensation is given for such services. But in the state of Maharashtra and Andhra Pradesh the staff nurses on night duty are paid Rs.20 per month as special allowance.

According to Vroom, the work role occupied by a person affects here working hours as well as her spending of leisure time. A person's job usually influences the community in which the lives, the way in which other members of the community respond to him and the amount of time she can spend with her children. The basic assumption is that the valence of a given work schedule for a person is an inverse function of the extent to which that work schedule restricts her ability to enjoy leisure activity. An enquiry on the hours spent in domestic care, leisure time available and the leisure time activities of the nurses has been made through personal interview. The interview throws some light on the relationship between the work schedule and job satisfaction of nurses. All the male nurses

(3) respond that they spend no time in domestic work but only two nurses respond that they partially bear the burden of domestic work. Those from joint families respond that all the time available other than duty hours at the hospital is spent in domestic work. As to the rest of the hours, it is reported that male nurses in the sample can take rest all the time other than their duty hours at the hospital. Five nurses respond that they snatch a rest of an hour or so but nothing can provide them the mental rest, relaxation or peace of mind. Nurses are house wives and mothers responsible for the peace and happiness of their families. But they themselves have no time to enjoy the family life.

As to the leisure time activities seventeen nurses report that they prefer to take rest and only complete rest when they have leisure time at their disposal. Other activities in the leisure hours are sewing, knitting, reading and writing, preparation of new recipes, sports and social work. Half of the existing nurses stick to the traditional leisure time activities of women like sewing, knitting, cooking etc. More than one–third of the nurses (107) regularly read religious, philosophical or spiritual literature for reducing mental strain and tension which they have to face during the working hours. Fifteen enlightened nurses try to keep their knowledge upto date by reading magazines and periodicals related to medical profession. It is really interesting to note that some of the nurses have high social consciousness and they make special efforts to improve their English as well. They look around with an open mind and want to use their leisure in some sort of creative work. Only two nurses speak of their leisure time activities for sports like badminton or tennis. They rarely attend any entertainment programmes even though they have a liking for music, dance and drama etc. Even when they are away from their routine life, the domestic responsibilities consume all their leisure and energy making it impossible to develop their hobbies. Moreover, odd and abnormal duty hours prevent them from enjoying the leisure. All the nurses agree that the position would not have been much different in the even of their accepting some other employment.

Inconvenient work schedule and long hours of work with a night duty of 12 hours may be less strainous with proper and regular rest intervals. Nurses doing a standing duty for long hours in the atmosphere of diseases under too much mental and physical strain, certainly need adequate rest breaks during the work day. The rest break can reduce the fatigue and refresh them for serving the patients again. Since nurses are not machines but human beings, some sort of mental relief like talking to friends and engaging themselves in some other thoughts, need to be provided to revitalise them intermittently. Nurses have no separate toilets to use and no resting rooms to relax during working hours and they find it difficult to have meals or tea while on duty. The work in wards becomes indefinite and monotonous and creates boredom and job dissatisfaction. According to Wyatt, Fraser and Stock (1929), "The amount of boredom experienced by an employee bears some relation to the conditions of work and it is less liable to arise when suitable rest pauses are introduced within the spell of work". The Secretary, Orissa Nursing Employees Association emphasises on the recreational facilities of nurses, like duty rooms, lavatories and adequate water supply facilities for the nursing staff during duty hours. The Nursing Staff do night shift duty and in the hospital wards continuously for eleven hours from 9.00 p.m. to 8.00 a.m. and greatly suffer for wants of lavatories. In the absence of duty rooms, they stay on the hospital varandahs even in winter nights.

Nurses in three medical college hospitals of Orissa are state Government employees. The rules regarding weekly rest, holidays and leave of different kinds prescribed by the Government of Orissa for its employees are applicable to them also. They do not press for more holidays and leave, but they have a few suggestions to make on the enforcement of these rules in view of the fact that in actual practice they only avail a very limited advantage of these rules. They are of the opinion that it is impossible to take a legitimate leave or holiday when some other employee is not available to act as a reliever. It is, therefore, necessary to increase the size of the nursing staff in a hospital to enable the existing staff to enjoy their holidays and leave as per rules. In fact, it would be a healthy practice if every nurse is asked to proceed on compulsory leave for one month in a year to take complete rest and attend to her health problems. Although the existing rules of Indian Nursing Council (INC) contain such provision, yet, it is not compulsorily enforced without reducing their allowances. They feel discriminated against in the matter of availing leave benefits. For instance, a clerk automatically avails himself of the Sunday as a holiday after availing a week long casual leave from Monday to Saturday, but a nurse has to report herself to duty at the end of her week's casual leave.

The General Conference of the International Labour Organisation (ILO) adopted the Nursing Personnel Recommendation on its 63rd session in 21st June, 1977. The Nursing Personnel Recommendation puts down specifically the expectations of the nurses throughout the world regarding their working time and periods of rest. They are as follows:

(VIII) Working Time and Rest Periods

(30) For the purpose of this Recommendation,

(a) the term "**normal hours of work**" means the number of hours fixed in each country by or in pursuance of laws or regulations, collective agreements or arbitration awards;

(b) the term "**over time**" means hours worked in excess of normal hours of work;

(c) the term "**on–call duty**" means periods of time during which nursing personnel are; at the work place or elsewhere, at the disposal of the employer, in order to respond to possible calls;

(d) the term "**inconvenient hours**" means hours worked on other than the normal working days and other than the normal working time of the country.

(31) The time during which nursing personnel are at the disposal of the employer–such as the time needed to receive and transmit instructions should be counted as working time for nursing personnel, subject of possible special provisions concerning on–call duty.

(32)

(1) The normal weekly hours of nursing personnel should not be higher than those set in the country concerned for workers for general.

(2) Where the normal working week of workers in general exceeds 40 hours, steps should be taken to bring it down, progressively, but as rapidly as possible, to that level for nursing personnel, without any reduction in salary.

(33)

(1) Normal daily hours of work should be continuous and not exceed eight hours, except where arrangements are made by laws and regulations, collective agreements, works rules or arbitration awards for flexible hours or a compressed week; in any case, the normal working week should remain within the limits set in the country concerned for workers in general.

(2) The working day, including overtime, should not exceed 12 hours.

(3) Temporary exceptions to the above provisions should be authorised only in case of special emergency.

(34)

(1) There should be mean breaks of reasonable duration.

(2) There should be rest breaks of reasonable duration included in the normal hours of work.

(35) Nursing personnel should have sufficient notice of working schedules to enable them to organise their personal and family life accordingly. Exceptions to these schedules should be authorised only in case of special emergency.

(36)

(1) Where nursing personnel are entitled to less than 48 hours of continuous weekly rest, steps should be taken to bring their weekly rest to that level.

(2) The weekly rest of nursing personnel should in no case be less than 36 uninterrupted hours.

(37)

(1) There should be as little recourse to overtime work, work at inconvenient hours and on–call duty as possible.

(2) Overtime and work on public holidays should be compensated by an addition to salary.

(38)

(1) Shift work should be compensated by an increase in remuneration which should not be less than that applicable to shift work in other employment in the country.

(2) Nursing personnel assigned to shift work should have a period of continuous rest of at least 12 hours between shifts.

(3) A single shift of duty divided by a period of unremunerated time (split shift) should be avoided.

(39)

(1) Nursing personnel should be entitled to, and required to take, a paid annual holiday of at least the same length as other workers in the country.

(2) Where the length of the paid annual holiday is less than four weeks for one year of service, steps should be taken to bring it progressively, but as rapidly as possible, to that level for nursing personnel.

(40) Nursing personnel who work in particularly arduous or unpleasant conditions should have benefit from a reduction of working hours and/or an increase in rest periods, without any decrease in total remuneration.

(41)

(1) Nursing personnel absent from work by reason of illness or injury should be entitled, for a period and in a manner determined by laws or regulations or by collective agreements to –

(a) Maintenance of the employment relationship and of rights deriving therefrom.

(b) Income security.

(2) The laws or regulations, or collective agreements, establishing sick leave entitlement should distinguish between –

(a) Cases in which the illness or injury is service–incurred;

(b) Cases in which the person concerned is not incapacitated for work but absence from work is necessary to protect the health of others ;

(c) Cases of illness or injury unrelated to work.

(42)

(1) Nursing personnel, without distinction between married and unmarried persons, should be assured the benefits and protection provided for in the Maternity Protection Convention (Revised), 1952 and the Maternity Protection Recommendation, 1952.

(2) Maternity leave should not be considered to be sick leave.

(3) The measures provided for in the Employment (women with Family Responsibilities) Recommendations, 1956 should not be applied in respect of nursing personnel.

(43) Decisions concerning the organisation of work, working time and rest periods should be taken in agreement or in consultation with freely chosen representatives or the nursing personnel or with organisations representing them.

They should bear, in particular, on

(a) the hours to be regarded as inconvenient hours,

(b) the condition is in which the exception to these provisions will be authorised,

(c) the conditions in which on–call duty will be counted as working time,

(d) the length of the rest breaks and the manner in which they are to be taken,

(e) the form and the amount of the compensation provided for the overtime, work on public holidays and shift work,

(f) working schedule, and

(g) the conditions to be considered as particularly arduous or unpleasant.

The General Conference of the International Labour Organisation, at the same time, made the following suggestions concerning practical application of the above recommendations :

(18)

(1) In the organisation of hours of work, every effort should be made, subject to the requirements of the service, to allocate shift work, overtime work and work at inconvenient hours equitably between nursing personnel, and in particular between permanent and temporary and between full time and part time personnel, and to take account as far as possible of individual preference and of special considerations regarding such matters as climate, transportation and family responsibilities.

(2) The organisation of hours of work for nursing personnel should be based on the need for nursing services rather than subordinated to the work pattern of other health service personnel.

(19)

(1) Appropriate measures to limit the need for overtime, for work at inconvenient hours and for on–call duty should be taken in the orgainsation of work, in determining the number and the use of staff and in scheduling hours of work; in particular, account should be taken of the need for replacing nursing personnel during absences or leave authorised by laws or regulations or collective agreements, so that the personnel who are present will not be over–burdened.

(2) Overtime should be worked on a voluntary basis, except where it is essential for patient care and sufficient volunteers are not available.

(20) The notice of working schedules should be given at least two weeks in advance.

(21) Any period of on–call duty during which nursing personnel are required to remain at the work place or the services of the nursing personnel are actually used should be fully regarded as working time and remunerated as such.

(22)

(1) Nursing personnel should be free to take their meals in places of their work–place.

(2) They should be able to take their rest breaks at a place other than their work–place.

(3) The time at which the annual holiday is to be taken should be determined in an equitable basis, due account being taken of family obligations, individual preferences and the requirements of the services.

Taking the present situation in the college hospitals of Orissa into consideration, it may be affirmed that there is a necessity for enforcing the recommendations of the General Conference of the ILO. These recommendations need be implemented in to far improving the working conditions of the nurses in regard to the night duty, rest pause and a place for rest pause etc.

Work Group

Work group is a vital factor to pass the working hours. In modern organisation like college hospitals a large number of employees are working together. A nurse cannot work in isolation, she is continuously associated with other nurses, supervisors, doctors, medical officers and class IV employees etc. Her work group influences her job satisfaction and productivity to a large extent.

Work groups must be attractive to their members to the extent to which the nature of the situation permits or requires interaction. The degree of attraction between any two members of the group should be directly related to the extent to which they interact with one another in course of the performance of their work. Every individual must get an opportunity to interact with other frequently in course of performance of his work. The situation itself should require or permit the workers to coaliate so as to create favourable job attitude among the employees. Newcomb hypothesises that interaction between members of the group is rewarding when it results in cognition of similar attitudes towards important and relevant objects. He says, "If a member of a group perceives other members as having similar attitudes towards relevant objects, he feels positive attraction towards the group and the job". Because similarity of attitudes permits the "ready caclculabilty of others behaviour" as well as "the validation of one's own orientation towards relevant objects".

Another variable which is said to affect the attractiveness of work group for its members is the degree to which they are accepted or valued by other group members. Bellows is of the opinion that, "The manner in which a new employee is accepted by and adjusts to his fellow workers may determine to a large extent his satisfaction with his job, employer, boss and the firm, his amount of production and even the length of time he remains with the company". Another point to be noted about the work group is that interaction between two members of the group should satisfy both, creating attraction towards each other and favourable attitude towards the job. Then only interaction has the consequence of facilitating the progress of each of the member towards attainment of his goals. Interdependence of goals is necessary. The interaction of the members should be co–operative, not competitive.

The nurses in college hospitals in the study are studied as members of the work group. Similarity of attitudes towards the job, patients, superiors and subordinates are expected from them. But the study reveals that there is a wide gap of understanding between these nurses and the nurses working in higher levels of management. A feeling of togetherness is not found in between Matrons, Assistant Matrons, and the Sisters and Staff Nurses. Only there are very few exceptions. For instance, all of them disapprove the high handed behaviour of doctors, visiting specialists and medical officers. Besides that, all of them agree on the urgent necessity of discipline the arrogant and unruly class IV employees. Enhancing the standard of medical care presupposes the coordination and co–operation among all categories of medical employees.

4.2 Physical Facilities

Physical facilities at work place of nurses are the most vital factor of working conditions. It depends upon several factors like Departmental lay out, Lighting and Ventilation, Cleanliness, Rest rooms, Messing, Sanitary blocks and Occupational health protections. Every employee expects the work place to be well lighted, ventilated and pleasantly coloured. The three medical college hospital buildings have been built according to the needs of the hospitals. The rooms are big enough to accommodate patients and have attached toilets. But the large inflow of patients make these spacious wards overcrowded so much so that the patients occupy every inch of the possible floor space available in the wards. The only remedy of this is to control the admission of patients. The accommodation of larger number of patients put a lot of physical strain on nurses and they face difficulties in the supervision of the wards as well as attending the patients properly.

In MKCG Medical College hospital, lighting and ventilation is satisfactory. In SCB and VSS Medical College hospitals, some blocks are in dilapidated condition. Patients and nurses are affected due to lack of proper lighting and ventilation. Dim light in work places puts pressure on the eye and increases fatigue. The nurses may have headache, eye pain, congestion around cornea, distraction from visual tasks and loss of concentration which may result from direct glare. Indirect glare from an intense light spot may cause blurring of vision. Reflected glare from shiny surfaces or dials can prevent perception of visual displays.

Cleanliness leads so Godliness. The work place must be clean, otherwise the biological agents in the work environment like viruses, rickettsia, bacteria, and parasites of various types may affect the individual's health. Wards are gradually kept clean, but the corridors, staircases and waiting rooms are shabby only because of the improper use made of them by the patients and their attendants or relatives. Treatment in medical college hospital is mostly free of charge. So the patients come from every nook and corner of the State to avail of the free service. They are unconcerned about the cleanliness of the blocks and corridors.

Adequate resting and messing facilities are the dire need of the nurses working for hours together in the company of sick people in order to relieve themselves of fatigue caused by overwork. Almost in all the three college hospitals, there are no separate rooms for the nurses. Those having nearby accommodation, relax and get refreshed at home. But persons coming from far off places just spend a few moments in the old–fashioned, dull and drab duty rooms and have the hurried meals. In view of the excessive pressure of work, spacious, airy, clean, pleasantly coloured rest rooms with furniture, light magazines, newspapers and other recreational facilities have become the prime necessity for the persons of this profession.

Occupational health protection is another necessity. They work for long hours in the unhealthy atmosphere of the sick and the diseased and are susceptible to infection. Particularly those who work in TB wards or in the wards accommodating patients with communicable diseases are exposed to greater degree of danger for their health. Similarly, nurses in mental hospitals have to live with continuous mental tension in dealing with the patients. Because of its peculiar nature, the nursing occupation needs special provisions for protection of health of the nurses. Regular medical checkup, provisions of adequate treatment, recoupment and rest, leave and other allowances, provision of nutritious diet etc. are the measures to be taken to protect their health. Nurses, working in hospitals are normally paid washing allowance for cleanliness which varies from state to state. Whereas the nurses serving under the Central Government are given an allowance of Rs. 15 per month, the Governments of Andhra Pradesh and Maharashtra pay @ Rs. 20 per month to the nurses serving under them. But there is no such provision in Orissa. Similarly, no special messing allowance is given to nurses in Orissa as is given to their counterparts in Maharashtra. Nurses in mental hospitals of Andhra Pradesh and Maharashtra receive a special allowance of Rs. 20 per month which of course, is enjoyed by the nurses of Orissa.

The major categories of environmental agents and conditions for workers in their work places are

(i) physical agents and conditions,
(ii) biological agents and conditions,
(iii) chemical agents, and
(iv) psychological factors.

The hazardous physical agents and conditions are unsatisfactory lighting conditions and exposure to heat and cold. Biological agents and conditions are viruses, rickettsia, bacteria and parasites of various types. Chemical agents like tonic chemicals and dusts lead to respiratory diseases like pulmonary fibrosis, obstructive long diseases, allergy and even cancer. Similarly shift work, speed and safety may adversely influence the health of the workers. Nurses should avoid such conditions to protect their health.

The general conference of the ILO in lst June, 1977 has made the following suggestions –

(44) Each member should endeavour to adopt laws and regulations on occupational health and safety to the special nature of nursing work and the environment in which it is carried out, and to increase the protection afforded by them.

(45) (1) Nursing personnel should have access to occupational health services operating in accordance with the provisions of the Occupational Health Services Recommendations, 1959.

(2) Where occupational health services have not yet been set up for all undertakings, medical care establishments employing nursing personnel should be among undertakings for which such services should be set up in the Ist instance.

(46) (1) Each member and the employers' and workers' organisations concerned should pay particular attention to the provisions of the protection of Workers' Health Recommendation, 1953 and endeavour to ensure its application to nursing personnel.

(2) All appropriate measures should be taken to prevent, reduce or eliminate risks to the health or safety of nursing personnel.

(17) (1) Nursing personnel should undergo medical examinations on taking up and terminating an appointment at regular intervals during their service.

(2) Nursing personnel regularly assigned to work in circumstances such that a definite risk to their health or to that of others around them exits or may be suspected should undergo regular medical examinations at intervals appropriate to the risk involved.

(3) Objectivity and confidentiality should be assured in examinations provided for in this paragraph; the examinations referred to should not be carried out

by doctors with whom they have a close working relationship.

(48) (1) Studies should be undertaken and kept upto date to determine special risks to which nursing personnel may be exposed in the exercise of their profession so that these risks may be prevented and compensated.

(2) For that purpose, cases of occupational accidents and cases of diseases recognised as occupational under laws or regulations concerning employment injury benefits, or liable to be occupational in origin, should be notified to the competent authority, in a manner to be prescribed by national laws or regulations in accordance with paragraphs with 14 to 17 of the protection of workers' health recommendation, 1953.

(49) (1) All possible steps should be taken to ensure that nursing personnel are not exposed to special risks. Where exposure to special risks is unavoidable, measures should be taken to minimise it.

(2) Measures such as the provision and use of protective clothing, immunisation, shorter hours, more frequent rest breaks, temporary removal from the risk or longer annual holidays should be provided for in respect to nursing personnel regularly assigned to duties involving special risks so as to reduce their exposure to these risks.

(3) In addition, nursing personnel who are exposed to special risks should receive financial compensation.

(50) Pregnant women and parents of young children whose normal assignment could be prejudicial to their health or that of their children should be transferred, without loss of entitlements, to work appropriate to their situation.

(51) The collaboration of nursing personnel and of organisations representing them should be sought in ensuring the effective application of provisions concerning the protection of the health and safety of nursing personnel.

(52) Appropriate measures should be taken for the supervision of the application of the laws and regulations and other provisions concerning the protection of the health and safety of nursing personnel.

For the practical application of the above suggestions, Recommendation 157 noticed out as follows.

(24) Nursing personnel in respect of whom special measures should be taken should include, in particular, personnel regularly exposed to radiations into anaestthetic substances and personnel in contact with infectious diseases or mental illness.

(25) Nursing personnel regularly exposed to ionising radiations should in addition enjoy the protection of the measures provided for in the Radiation Protection Convention and Recommendation, 1960.

(26) Work to which pregnant women or mothers of young children should not be assigned should include:

(a) as regards women covered by paragraph 5 of the Maternity Protection Recommendation, 1952, the types of work enumerated therein;

(b) generally, work involving exposure to ionising radiation or anesthetic substances or involving contact with infectious diseases.

(27) In order to ensure continuity in the acquisition of rights and the provision of benefits steps should be taken to coordinate such private supplementary schemes as exist with each other and with stationary schemes.

(28) In order to ensure that nursing personnel receive the compensation for illness contracted as a result of their work, members should, by laws or regulations –

(a) Prescribe a list establishing a presumption of occupational origin in respect of certain diseases when they contracted by nursing personnel, and revise the list periodically in the light of scientific and technical developments affecting nursing personnel.

(b) Complement that list by a general definition of occupational diseases or by other provision enable nursing personnel to establish the occupational origin of disease not presumed to be occupational by virtue of the list.

The General Conference of the ILO in the same session, passed a resolution concerning the application of certain International Labour standards to nursing personnel, in which it noted, in particular, that the Employment Injury Benefits Convention, 1964, covered all employees, the exclusion of public servants being possible only where they are covered by schemes providing equivalent benefits, and that the scope of Maternity Protection Convention (Revised), 1952 included "establishment for the treatment and care of the sick (and) infrim", and it appealed to all member countries to ensure that the provisions of these instruments are fully applied in practice to nursing personnel.

An employee spends the best part of his day at the work–place for which payment is made. But it is important to look to the overall welfare of the employees rather than considering the monetary reward alone. A feeling of team spirit and oneness may be created by improving the standard of living of the nurses which will help them in developing their personality as responsible citizen and give full scope for the development of their aspirations. Welfare activities like sports, culture and various types of competition need be organised under the overall charge of the welfare officers.

4.3 Job Satisfaction

Job Satisfaction or job content refers to pleasantness or unpleasantness of the work to employee. It expresses the level of agreement between one's expectations of the job and rewards that the job provides. Since job content involves expectations, it is related to equity, the psychological contact and motivation. Further, the number and nature of functions performed by an employee has a tremendous impact on the employee's job satisfaction. Favourable factors of job–content are wages, promotional opportunities, level and status of the employee, specialisation, Control of over work and job security etc. Similarly, unfavourable factors of job content are bad supervision, poor decision making power and confusion delegation leading to job dissatisfaction. The nature of work in the various posts of nurses is interesting and meaningful. The patient who happens to be a human being is the focus of all the activities in the profession and that itself makes their work exciting attractive and fascinating. The sample nurses, therefore, agree that their work is never boring or monotonous. Extending nursing care to sick and relieving them of their pains and agony give them immense satisfaction which cannot be measured in terms of money.

The issue of wages or remuneration determining worker's job satisfaction is not free from controversy. Economists are prone to stress the importance of the size of the pay in determining worker's job satisfaction and probability of his remaining in the job. Social scientists are associated with the human relations movement typically view economic factors as highly over emphasised and stress the importance of the satisfaction and social ego needs. Vroom says, "When workers are asked to rank different aspects of the work–role in terms of their importance, wages tend to be rated as less important than security and opportunity for advancement. Rather company and management are considered to be more important than job content, supervision, the social aspects of the job, communication, working conditions and benefits. However, when they are asked to describe what makes them satisfied or dissatisfied with their jobs, wages are found to be the most frequent source of dissatisfaction but it is the least important source of satisfaction for the nurses (Table 23).

It is noticed from the resolutions passed by Orissa Nursing Employees Association that the nurses in Orissa are deprived of several allowances which their counterparts under the Central Government and several other state Government are enjoying for the past decades. These include Uniform allowance, Washing allowance, Nursing allowance, Messing allowance, Special allowance, Employees Staff Insurance Scheme (ESIS) allowance, Ration allowance, Stitching allowance, Non–Government Officials (NGOs) Clinic allowance and Compensatory salary etc.

Table 23 reveals the wage structure of nurses form the lowest to the highest rank. It is really disheartening to note that the Nursing Superintendent or a Principal gets a Class–II scale after a continuous service and sacrifice of more than 25 years and a Staff Nurse gets much less in comparism to that of her counterparts elsewhere.

Table 23: Wage Structure (Pay Scale) of Nurses

Rank	*Designation*	*Pay Scale*
1.	Staff Nurse	Rs. 4500–7000
2.	Asstt. Matron Nursing Sister	Rs. 4750–8000
3.	Matron/ Nursing Supdt. Gr.II	Rs. 5300–8300
4.	Chief Matron/ Nursing Supdt. Gr.I	Rs. 6500–10500
5.	Nursing Supdt./ Principal Tutor/Principal	Rs. 8000–13500

Source: Directorate of Health and Family Welfare, Government of Orissa.

Organisation may be described as a hierarchy of roles. Role occupants may remain in the same role throughout their organisational membership or they may be promoted to a role involving greater wages, power and status. The opportunities for promotion offered to members of the organisationare highly variable and often assured to have a marked effect on job satisfaction because a position at a higher level in the same organisation typically involves changes in Supervision, co–workers' job content and pay. A person's evaluation of his present position directly affects the expectations regarding promotion. Ample promotional opportunities assure an employee of full utilisation and development of his skills and abilities and a chance to grow. A promotion earned in a service may be an excellent psychological and motivational factor for the employees to satisfy higher order needs like esteem, status, self–actualisation and fulfilment.

Out of 379 nurses interviewed in the three medical college hospitals, 363 have complained of their difficulties in getting a promotion in their service career. It appears there is total dissatisfaction on the question of promotional opportunities. A trained nurse is first appointed as a staff nurse who may not expect to be a Nursing Sister after 25 years of service (Table 7). A promotion to the post of Nursing Sister is a rare phenomenon and it at all it comes, it usually becomes the first and last promotion in the life of a nurse. Only five of them have been promoted to the post of Asst. Matron and three to the post of Matron. The number of posts at that level in the organisation is too much limited to satisfy the cadre. This is a very depressing situation which is naturally detrimental to any scheme of development and progress. This feeling of indifference and depression is well reflected in the questions put by a young staff nurse, "why should we work more and better? Why should we keep our knowledge upto date? Why should we take the trouble of gaining higher qualification? Why is there no monetary reward for the extra labour we put in?"

Nurses of multiple categories are also one of the important reasons of the lack of promotional opportunities in the cadre. After completing a course, a nurse is appointed in some hospital which may or may not be a teaching institution. Her appointment and cadre determination are only done by the Government and the nurses have no choice to make in this regard. A nurse working in a non–teaching institution (any hospital) cannot be promoted to a higher post easily or cannot get a promotion to a teaching institution as it happens in case of nurses working in the three medical college hospitals of Orissa. Secondly, a promotion in most of the cases is associated with transfer which poses many problems like security, accommodation and separation from the family etc. Thirdly, another obstacle is associated with the discriminatory policy of the Government in favour of Scheduled Castes and Scheduled Tribe candidates. Consequently, more qualified and efficient nurses from Brahmin, Kayastha and other higher castes are debarred from getting their promotion in due course. It creates frustration, agony and dissatisfaction among the nurses belonging to higher classes and they feel psychologically sick to work under a junior. Fourthly, the system of confidential reports of the matron in the matter of promotion sometimes leaves much scope for favouritism.

In the deliberations of Orssia Nursing Employees, Association (ONEA) in its meeting held at Berhampur (Ganjam) on 26th and 27th of May, 1990 had made the following recommendations on promotional opportunities.

(1) Several cadres of nurses and their types such as in non–teaching institution should be demolished and promotions should be given irrespective of cadre.

(2) Seniority, sincerity in work, extraordinary skill and special or additional qualifications must receive proper weightage.

(3) Before giving a promotion, every day work and performance for several years should be revised impartially.

(4) There should be no discrimination on the basis of sex.

(5) Promotion should not be dependent on the caste of candidates.

(6) It the promoted nurse is transferred to another place proper arrangements regarding accommodation personal security, education or children should be made. If she is married, her husband should also be transferred to that place, if possible, to avoid disruption of the family life.

(7) To reduce favouritism, the procedure of allotment of promotions on the basis of confidential reports should be changed and departmental or wardwise examinations similar to bank examinations should be conducted for competing candidates.

The General Conference of the ILO in its Recommendation No. 157 concerning employment and conditions of work and life of nursing personnel has made the following suggestions for the career development of the nurses

(21) (1) Measures should be taken to offer nursing personnel reasonable career prospects by providing for a sufficient varied and open range of possibilities of professional advancement, leadership positions in direct and supporting nursing care, the administration of nursing services, nursing education and research and development in the field of nursing and a grading and remuneration structure recognising the acceptance of functions involving increased responsibility and required greater technical skill and professional adjustment.

(2) These measures should be taken to give nursing personnel advice and guidance on career prospects and as appropriate, on re–entry into nursing after a period of interruption.

(22) These measures should also give recognition to the importance of functions involving direct relations with patients and the public.

(23) In determining the level at which nursing personnel reentering the profession after an interruption of its practice should be employed, account should be taken of previous nursing experience and the duration of the interruption.

45 (24) (1) Nursing personnel wishing to participate in programmes of continuing education and training and capable of doing so called be given the necessary facilities.

(2) These facilities might consist in the grant of paid or unpaid educational leave, adaptation of hours of work, and payment of study or training costs; whatever possible, nursing personnel should be granted paid educational leave in accordance with the paid Education Leave Convention, 1974.

(3) Employers should provide staff and facilities for in-service training of nursing personnel, preferably at the workplace.

The General Conference, in the Annex to the Recommendation 157, made the following suggestions concerning practical application of the above recommendation:

(11) Where the possibilities of professional advancement are limited as a result of the manner in which nursing services in general are concerned, measures might be taken to facilitate access to studies leading to qualifications for other health professions.

(12) (1) Measures should be taken to establish systems of classification and of scales of remuneration which provide possibilities of professional advancement on the basis of the classification of the level of functions.

(2) These systems should be sufficiently open to provide an incentive for nursing personnel to pass from one level to another.

(3) The promotion of nursing personnel should be based on equitable criteria and take account of experience and demonstrated ability.

(13) Increase in remuneration should be provided for, at every level, by reference to the development of experience and ability.

(14) (1) Measures should be taken to encourage nursing personnel to make the greatest possible use of their knowledge and their qualifications in their work.

(2) The responsibilities effectively assumed by nursing personnel and the competence shown by them should be continuously reviewed so as to ensure remuneration and possibilities of advancement or promotion corresponding thereto.

(15) (1) Periods of paid education leave should be considered to the periods of work for the purpose of entitlement to social benefits and other rights deriving from the employment relationship.

(2) As far as possible, periods of unpaid educational leave for the purpose of additional education and training should be taken into consideration in the calculation of seniority particularly as regards remuneration and pension rights.

These are the proposals to be followed by national and state government in context of the nurses. But it is not implemented in Orissa.

Apart from the problems of wage and promotional opportunities, another problem that hinders the job satisfaction is the problem of transfer. A transfer normally brings in its trail some problems and changes which a nurse very often fails to cope with and in most cases they give up their promotion just to avoid a transfer. Transfer results in a lot of dislocations in their family life which they are not prepared to accept. Unless they take it as a fact of life and refrain from becoming sick of it, it would continue to pose a big problem. Most of the nurses of SCB Medical College hospital temperamentally oppose to any transfer because of the better educational facilities available at Cuttack and the distinct prestige they enjoy as members of the biggest and oldest college hospital of the state. About 90 per cent of the unmarried nurses of three medical college hospitals are not prepared to go on transfer because of their attachment to their home towns and their total unpreparedness to face problems associated with transfer. Similarly, 30 per cent of the total number of nurses who are ambitious and enlightened take the plea that these college hospitals are the best to acquire knowledge and skill in the field and hence they are not willing to leave on transfer. Almost 99 per cent of the nurses in three medical college hospitals are averse of a transfer to rural areas because of lack of modern amenities like water supply, electricity, sanitary arrangements, educational facilities for the children, recreational facilities and facilities for transport and communication etc.

There is a positive relationship between the level or status of the worker and the satisfaction he/she derives from the job. It is interesting to know the opinion of the selected nurses regarding the status they enjoy. As to the level of status of job in society as a whole, 99 per cent of the nurses are of the view that their profession does not get its due recognition, respect and status from society. But in contrast to it, they are so much dedicated and attached to their work that none of them is interested for any attractive alternative. All the nurses have the unanimous demand for positive steps to be taken to enhance the status of the nursing community and realise and restore their dignity through a campaign and through the mass communication media. Higher level and status may increase the job satisfaction and boost up the working life of nursing personnel to some extent.

Specialisation is another determinant of job satisfaction which vary with the degree of specialisation in the job content. Greater specialisation increases repetitiveness of the job leading to a reduction in the job satisfaction. The effects of repetitive work, received considerable attention during the 1920s in the work of Industrial Fatigue Research Board in Great Britain. A large number of studies have been conducted both in Laboratory and industrial settings on the determinants and consequences of monotony and boredom in the work. The major conclusions of these are studies are summerised by Wyatt, Fraser and Stock as follows.

The amount of boredom experienced bears some relation to the conditions of work. It is liable to arise as follows –

(a) When the form of activity is changed at suitable times within the spell of work,

(b) When the operative are paid according to output instead of time worked,

(c) When the work is conceived as a series of self contained tasks rather than as an indefinite and apparently interminable activity.

(d) When the operatives are allowed to work in compact social groups rather than as isolated units.

(e) When suitable rest pauses are introduced within the spell of work.

A job which calls for a single operation or a very few operations to be performed over and over again reduces job satisfaction. One of the reasons for this can be the physiological process of fatigue. Continuous activation of a muscle results in a decreasee in the probability amplitude of the response. It appears reasonable to assume that performing the same operation over and over again would be more fatiguing than performing different operations because it would involve the use of different muscles, but many of the repetitive jobs which are disliked are not fatiguing in the usual sense of the term. It is not the amount of physical effort which the workers require but its **"sameness"** which creates boredom. After repeated performance of an activity the subject becomes psychologically satiated for the activity. Even though initially it might have been pleasant, the repetition of an activity results in deterioration characterised by efforts to change the activity, followed by a complete intolerance for it. Therefore, it is necessary to make a job less repetitive by increasing the number of operations which the worker performs or by increasing the frequency with which he can change from one operation to another. Job enlargement refers to increase in the number of operations to be performed which typically increased the frequency with which they can change from one operation to another. On the other hand in case of job rotation, which is another way of decreasing the repetitiveness of work, the content of a single work role remains the same, although the worker is enabled to move periodically from one work role to another. The effect, as far as repetitiveness is concerned, is to increase the total number of operations that the worker performs over along period but not to increase the frequency with which he can alternate from one operation to another. In the present study, effort is made to find out whether the nurses rated their work roles as monotonous and boring and if so, does the Government take any step to reduce the repetitiveness in their work by designing job enlargement on job rotation programmes.

Nurses have specific duties and responsibilities on different posts. Since their job is of a specialised nature, it may not be repetitive, monotonous and boring. The work roles are large enough which does not necessitate further job enlargement. It is gathered that no job rotation programmes are undertaken by the government purposefully, but transfer from one ward to another or from one department to another is not unusual. This automatically involves the process of job rotation. On the other hand, this sort of change of work becomes pleasurable because they are exposed to different types of patients, ailments and nursing pattern. They get a chance to learn new things with their new work roles. Sometimes they welcome a transfer from one to another work with the hope of avoiding transfer. A very small number of nurses prefer to work in one and the same ward continuously with a view to acquiring deep and intensive knowledge through their continuous work exposure with the patients of a particular category and ultimately win the admiration of the superiors for the same. That may also lead to innovative suggestions that may improve the overall working of the hospital conditions.

A generalist or a specialist may be a ticklish question. But the age of generalists in the health sciences is gone with all their advantages and disadvantages. It is the age of specialists and it has become a fact of life. Specialisation strengthens mental faculties and expands one's intellectual horizon. It helps in the acquisition of knowledge and skill, analyses and synthesises existing facts and generates new knowledge and wisdom. The scholars, the intellectuals, the innovative genius–all the products of specialisation. The scope of specialisation in any fields sets the standard of excellence and gives an added importance to the area. Specialised aspects of the profession improve the quality, make it distinctly prestigious and keep the profession on the move thus enabling it to face newer challenges and finding out inventive and innovative solution to them. It also increases efficiency and striking individuality in technique and approach.

The purview of specialisation in any field is the symbol if its excellence and quality. An inclination towards scholastic contemplation through the process of specialisation propagates the professional viability. A scholarly attitude inculcated in the course of specialisation stimulates multidimensional growth of productivity. Hence it injects a quest for better service of quality care. It is a matter of pride that the nursing profession can boast of specialists in its cadre who are trend setting performers in all spheres of nursing. But it is a paradox that there exists a handsome dearth of appropriate vacancies to absorb them. Thus, the nursing manpower remains utilised. This can be attributed to the absence of a proper recruitment culture. There is lacuna in the recruitment policies which has made the posts of specialists virtually non–existent. After obtaining a series of degrees one can attain the level of specialisation because various ongoing schemes only offer different course of specialisation.

The educational units in nursing have limited opportunities for specialisation, but barring a few exceptional cases their utilisation also leaves much to be desired. A specialised nurse trained in a particular discipline often finds herself placed in quite another area and her knowledge and skills remain utilised and thus wasted. Lack of courage determination and allied situations refrain the nurses to protest or resist such anomalies. Nursing is "**service to people**" and quality of one's service is directly proportional to the quality of one's preparation. If the present practice continues, the seriousness, the dynamism, the capacity to monitor one's action and one's intellectual response would reach a dead end. Taking into account the contemporary standard consciousness the competence of the trade must be developed in view of the fact that improvement in the performance profile happens to be the testimony to their professional quality.

Control over work method and control over work place have to be taken into account while determining an employee's job satisfaction. Pioneers in the field of management like Taylor, Frank and Lillian Gilbreth believe that workers who actually perform the job should not be permitted to decide how that job should be done and that planning of the job is a highly complex activity that requires the application of special techniques and so it should be separated form doing the job. The job can be entrusted to the workers but the method of it should be decided upon by the management. But viteles criticises the basic assumption of Taylor and Gilberth and emphasises that the best way of doing the work and depriving the worker of control over his own methods of work had negative consequences on worker's satisfaction.

According to Vroom, "The pace at which worker performs his job may be regulated either mechanically or socially,. but inability to control one's own pace of work is highly detrimental to worker satisfaction". Taking these observations on the nurses into account it can be said that their work is not related to machines, but to animate human beings which have emotions, feelings, and motives. Nurses, therefore, cannot use the same method of work and behaviour during the treatment of patients. They have to deal differently depending upon their experience, skill and needs of patients. Some of the nurses are of the opinion that it is impossible for the management to decide the work–method and work–pace for their type of job. Once the general frame work of duties are decided, a nurse has the freedom of determining her own method and speed of work within that frame work.

Generally an individual derives job satisfaction provided the work is within the skills and abilities of the worker. The over–worked nurse may not realise job satisfaction. A musician is for music, an artist must paint, a poet must write if he is to be ultimately happy. What a man can be must be. This is called "**self–actualisation**". The unsatisfied need for self–actualisation certainly affects her job satisfaction adversely.

Job security is an indirect determinant of job satisfaction. Usually an individual requires two types of security, *i.e.,* safety in work place and security of employment. Night duty and change of working hours from one shift to another may cause certain dislocations in the work–place. The Secretary, ONES laments in an interview that, "Nurses are always exposed to very awkward situations during night duty caused by unsocial and antisocial elements. The medical premises witness continuous disturbances by undesirable elements which brings psychological demoralisation to a female nurse". Appointment of security guards, therefore, are very vital for the safety and security of the nurses in the work–place. Secondly, security of the job is associated with confirmation of service. Generally an individual is initially employed by an organisation or the Government on a temporary basis. The Government observe the work for a specified period and confirm the incumbents on satisfactory performances. According to Vroom, "Job security is usually the most important aspect of work role according to common employee when he is asked to rank different aspects of his work role in terms of their importance". Job security brings permanence to a job which results in continuous receipt of fixed income on a fixed date enabling the employee to satisfy his numerous wants and gain material satisfaction. Job security and safety needs are second order of priority next only to physiological needs and are directly related to the job satisfaction of a worker. But unfortunately 70 per cent of nurses have not yet been confirmed in their services which gives rise to dissatisfaction. Viewed from the angle of the parameters discussed it may be inferred that the nurses are far from deriving job satisfaction from their services and some steps need be taken in this direction in order to insulate this invaluable service against the corrosion of standards, efficiency and high morals.

4.4 Supervision, Decision–making and Communication Gap

Supervision and delegation of authority are two interlinked indirect determinants of working conditions. Putnum, an enthusiastic proponent of this view point, had studied the results of the programme of interviewing in the famous Hawthrone works of the Western Electric Company and had remarked as follows.

"Finally the comments from employees have convinced us that the relationship between first line supervisors and the individual workman is of more important in determining the attitude, morale, general happiness and efficiency of that employee than any other single factor". In the context of nurses, it means that the relationship between the different levels of management like Matron, Sister, Staff Nurses etc. in the college hospital organisations must be harmonious, friendly and mutually faithful to create favourable job attitudes in all the employees. The immediate supervisor's attitude towards the job influences the worker's attitude and creativity to a large extent.

According to Vroom, "Supervisors can be characterised in the terms of the degree to which they are considerate of the desires of their subordinates". An employee–oriented supervisor is more considerate to his subordinates. His acts facilitate the attainment of rewards or avoidance of punishments by his subordinates. He establishes a supportive personal relationship with this subordinates, takes a personal interest in them and understands when mistakes are committed on the other hand, a production oriented supervisor views his subordinates as instruments to get the work done and is concerned primarily with achieving a high level of production.

Vroom further adds, "one of the basic assumptions of those associated with human relations is that persons obtains satisfaction from influencing decision and controlling their work environment". Terms such as group decision, democratic leadership and participative supervision, all of which have an important place in the literature on human relations, refer to supervisory styles which permit subordinates a substantial degree of influence on decisions which affect them. There is considerable evidence that the satisfaction of subordinates is positively associated with the degree to which they are permitted an opportunity to participate in decision making.

Information on the existing supervisory behaviour in college hospitals have been collected by personal interviews. It is found that comparatively lower levels of management are employee oriented, considerate and quite understanding. For example, there is supportive relationship between Sisters and Staff Nurses. Sisters are the experienced Staff Nurses of yester years and promoted to the rank after a substantially long record of service. A sister also cannot perform her duty effectively without complete and voluntary co–operation of the Staff Nurses. But the relationship between Sister Matron and Assistant Matron is less than cordial. Matrons and Assistant Matrons always try to extract high level of work from the nurses without undertaking the grievances of their subordinates. It appears as if there is large communication gap and lack of understanding between these two levels management which further worsens situation. Sometimes this lack of undertaking, co–operation and co–ordination bring chaos and confusion in the nursing community.

Surprisingly, it is found that nurses pay a very little thought to decision making aspect of their working conditions. In almost all the three medical college hospitals nobody except two is willing to participate in management and in the process of decision making. In SCB Medical College hospital two nurses have a desire to participate in the management. Five of them viewed that they have to equip themselves with many things before they participate in management. Seven of them suggest that along with the doctors and experts their leader need be properly posted with facts before the opening of new wards or hospitals to boost up their status in society.

Better communication is necessary for better supervision and decision making. Supervision, decision making and communication are interacting factors to ensure better working conditions of nurses. Davis defines communication "as the passing of information and also the understating from one person to another". It is a sharing of thoughts and the process by which a manager (or any supervisor) learns to manage his work. A person can initiate the process but may not complete it. It is completed by a receiver. It means that communication is a two way process. The purpose of communication is to supply the information necessary for job performance and active co–operation. In other words, communication provides the means whereby a plan can be implemented and action co–ordinated towards the common goal. It is a means whereby the members of the organisation can be motivated to execute such plans willingly and effectively. The management can perform its functions, like planning, organising, directing, co–ordinating and controlling and get the work done by the employees through effective communication.

Usually a nurse receives some information about the work during the course of the their training and the practical knowledge has to be gained through work experience only. New entrants learn by trial and error method. A few senior and experienced nurses held the new entrants and carry out the job in cooperation. Communication, being a two–way process, can never be completed by the nurse alone. According to learned, Ulrishc and Booz, "good communication exists where anyone in the organisation is free to contact whoever can help him with this problem and if the members are restricted to formal channels of communication only, they become frustrated". Not only the staff nurses but matrons also feel the existence of communication gap between themselves and their boss. Any change in the policy or introduction of new rules and regulations relating to the services of the nursing personnel on work in the hospitals come to the Matrons suddenly in the form of Government Resolution for immediate implementation. They do not get any opportunity to convey their reactions difficulties to the Government. The nature of their work is most uncertain which requires increased information flow in order to maintain a comparable level of performance. They also need a feed back about their performance to know how well they are meeting the organisational goals and enhancing their image with a feeling of success. They accept effective channels of communication to be developed in the organisation which could provide them information on items like working conditions, supervisory relationship, operating rules, fringe benefits and policies which affect them and their work directly.

4.5 Unions and Collective Bargaining

Nurses' Unions or their collective bargaining power is the most vital and indirect determinant of working conditions. Strong Union and its bargaining strength determine the conditions and facilities of work. At present three unions of nurses are working at the Central level : (1) **All India Government Nurses Federation (AIGNF)**, (2) **Trained Nurses' Union (TNU)** and (3) **Trained Nurses' Association of India (TNAI)**. Besides, there are two State level unions, namely (1) **Orissa Nursing Employee's Association (ONEA)**, and (2) **Trained Nurses' Association of India, Orissa Branch**. For the first time in 1974 an unrecognised association namely All Orissa Nursing Association was formed which was subsequently recognised on 25th September, 1981 as the **"Orissa Nursing Employees Association"**.

All nurses except the Gazetted nursing personnel are members of ONEA. But there is no clear–cut division of watertight compartments between the membership of ONEA and TNAI. All the problems of nursing community like creation of posts, confirmation, promotion prospects, job security and service facilities etc. are dealt with by this association which takes up these issues with the government from time to time for their redressal. With mounting problems the nurses have never gone on strike nor do they think of such a course of action in future. Their services being very essential can never be suspended with a view to securing some personal gains. Duty comes first in their order of preference and such compromising and elastic attitude of the union has earned for itself the unique distinction of being an association for service and sacrifice. However, ONEA is not as strong as the association of nurses in Karnataka where they have succeeded in establishing a separate directorate for them. Their bargaining power has thus enhanced their job security. The qualitative strength of the nursing union, therefore, depends upon its bargaining power.

The employer's scope of authority in respect of administrative powers and economic stability is much wider than that of the employees. The employer determines their activities, status, level of achievement and the most important, price of labour which is conducive for him. The concept of equality and democracy goes against the employee in such a situation. To correct the imbalance of authority and status, the worker ought to come together in an organisation of their own and deal with the employer on equal terms. They are to unite and make collective efforts to improve their working as well as social conditions. Opportunity of collective bargaining provides the psychological support, self confidence, feeling of dignity and equality.

As regards participation, Recommendations 157, ILO contain following suggestions.

(19) (1) Measure should be taken to promote the participation of nursing personnel in the planning and its decisions concerning national health policy in general and concerning their profession in particular at all levels, in a manner appropriate to national conditions.

(2) In particular

(a) qualified representatives of nursing personnel, or of organisations representing them, should be associated with the elaboration and application of policies and general principles regarding the nursing profession, including those regarding education and training and practice of the profession;

(b) conditions of employment and work should be determined by negotiations between the employers' and workers' organisations concerned;

(c) the settlement of disputes arising in connection with the determination of terms and conditions of employment should be sought through negotiation between the parties or through independent and impartial machinery, such as mediation, conciliation and voluntary arbitration, with a view to make it unnecessary for the organisations representing nursing personnel to have recourse to such other steps as are normally open to organisations of other workers in defence of their legitimate interests.

(d) in the employing establishment, nursing personnel or their representative should be associated with decisions relating to their professional life, in a manner appropriate to the question at issue.

(20) Representative of nursing personnel should be assured the protection provided for in the Workers' Representatives Convention on Recommendation, 1971".

In the annex of the above Recommendation 157, suggestions regarding practical application of policy concerning nursing services and nursing personnel have been given. The relationship between nursing personnel and other categories of health personnel are made in consultation with the employers' and workers' organisation concerned. However, a balanced organisational set up is necessary to strike out a balance between Authority and Trade union. But in Orissa the trade union has no such formidable role due to weak bargaining power. This bargaining power is weak only because of excessive workload, domestic pressure and predominance of females in the profession.

4.6 Living Conditions

A successful homelife is a corollary of a successful worklife. It is, therefore, the responsibility of the employer to take both homelife and worklife into account and provide ideal working and living conditions. Organisation means to help the people to attain their goals where an individual only spends a specific part of a day for daily bread. But for the remaining part of the day, he may be a member of the family, a student of educational institution, loyal citizen of a nation, a taxpayer of the corporation and a member of a political and social organisation. A nurse is employed for her specific ability or skill, but it is often observed that skill or ability is directly linked with the background of the nurses. Because worklife and homelife are so much interlinked with each other that each affects the other to a large extent. Davis supports the above view point while describing the nature of the people and the basic assumption of a **"whole person".**

A study of their living conditions is necessary to understand the problems of the nurses which is another important part in life. The determinants of living conditions are family set–up, homelife, accommodation and environment. As discussed earlier in the previous chapter, most of the nurses have accepted the job out of economic necessity which reflects their family types, family heads, educational status of family members and family size etc. Family is the place for household activities. An individual born into a family is expected to do some sacrifice which sometimes compels the nurses to work outside. Families of the nurses are classified into two groups—**nuclear family and joint family.**

In modern times the nuclear family is often found in the society due to the impact of modernisation, urbanisation and socio–economic changes in society. Nuclear family consists of the husband, wife and the children. But now a days it is called extended family because it is consisted of father, mother, father–in–law, mother–in–law, sister–in–law, non–adult cousin or a paying guest student. For the purpose of present study, unmarried nurses staying alone or with room–mates in rented rooms for the purpose of employment are regarded as members of nuclear family. On the other hand, the joint family consists of father–in–law, mother–in–law, brother–in–law, and their wives and the children in addition to nurse herself. For the purpose of present survey, an unmarried nurse living with her parents' family, which is joint family, is regarded as a member of joint family. The study reveals that 70 per cent of nurses belong to the nuclear family group and 26 per cent belong to joint family and the rest have nobody at all to love and be loved as family or relatives. They render motherly or sisterly love to the patients. For them hospital is their home and everything of their life.

Most of the nurses come from lower class or middle class families. It is, therefore, difficult to cope with the home work and work outside for them. Only few such women have the income as well as understanding and sympathy from the family which can ensure some rest and leisure for their staff improvement or enable them to adjust the patterns of social interactions demanded by their jobs with the demands of the home.

"The change in attitude to women working outside the home or participating in public life has been slow and uneven, because it is related to deep rooted prejudices about a women's inherent attitudes and capacities, her proper sphere of work and man–women relationships. A woman, primarily associated with the home, is expected to look after domestic chores and her typical roles are those of a house wife and mother. In cultural understanding of the people, home making like child rearing and child–bearing is identified with females. Whether women work in the fields, factories or mines, at construction sites or in white collar jobs, all of them are expected to be home makers in the same manner as woman who confine themselves exclusively to home making. Their role in the outside world has not yet been accepted at the same level as that of the men's.

The teaching profession and medicine are considered respectable for women in as much as they do not conflict with traditional family norms. Nursing, on the other hand, though in conflict with feminine roles, involves contact with impure objects, male patients and doctors, odd hours of work and has still not attained the same degree of acceptability among the middle classes except in few regions and communities. The Bible emphasises certain qualities of a woman such as her capacity to work, caring for her family, kindness and charity for the needy outside the home etc. Christianity does not emphasize marriage as a women's sole destiny. She has an independent moral entity and responsibility.

Further, the trend in labour market shows a decline in the number of Christian nurses in the profession and gradual increase in the number of nurses from other religions who have now come forward to take up the job. In the middle class from which most of the nurses come, the roles and spheres of activities of men and women are sharply demarcated. Economically they are weak. Necessarily, the men and the women folk divide among themselves the labour they contribute in earning their bread. Though the women are primarily saddled with the responsibility or rearing the children they have an economic role to play to supplement the income of their man folk in the family. The locality, educational level, economic level and extent to modernisation determine the division of labour and the nature of work to be performed by the women. As regards the facilities of sanitation, there is no problem for the nurses within the hospital campus. Hospitals are furnished with sanitary blocks. There is problem in case of nurses who remain outside. 40 per cent of them have sanitary facilities of bath rooms, latrine and water tap. But 60 per cent of nurses (remaining outside) face the inconveniences of sharing common latrine and fetching water from a distance etc.

Similarly from the point of view of work load in the family, it is found that only 14 per cent of nurses have whole time servants 21 per cent have part–time servants and the rest 65 per cent have no servants at all. The servants are employed for cleaning utensils, washing clothes, cleaning grain and getting it milled, cooking and looking after the children and other sundry duties. In VSS hospital, Burla, 92 per cent have either wholetime or part–time servants possibly due to easy availability of working hands at lower wages. Out of 379 nurses, 111 nurses could not afford to pay for servants due to economic hardship. Particularly all of them are the single earning member of the family. It is quite natural because nearly all these nurses accepted job due to economic compulsion and obviously they cannot spend their salaries for personal comfort or luxury. Some are not able to adjust with the habits of the servants and so they do their own work without depending on them.

There is a saying that **"Cleanliness leads to Godliness".** Healthy surrounding, atmosphere and locality make a man happy and provide consistent incentive to work hard. In fact, their surrounding lacks minimum possible environmental perfection. Considering their living conditions, particularly those who have got accommodation in SCB Medical College hospital, Cuttack, it may be said that it is far from satisfactory. The quarters are neither regularly white washed nor repaired. During rainy season most of quarters leak and get soaked. On the onset of the evening, antisocial elements and hooligans regularly make the place unsafe for living. That also tells upon their moral and work efficiency. The surrounding of their residences is crowded and polluted by patients and their attendants. In two other medical college hospitals the situation is slightly better only because of the recent construction of quarters. Although there is regular washing and cleaning of hospital campus, still then it is unhygienic due to misuse of patients and their attendants. Looking into their living and working conditions may be concluded that it is far from satisfaction which contradicts the hypothesis.

Chapter 5
Nursing Services in the Days Ahead

5.1 Retrospect

Health is the birth right of an individual. The concept of health as a basic right of social justice which has to be attained by the efforts of the individuals and communities and by selected organised health services. The Bhore Committee (1946), Shetty Committee (1953), Mudaliar Committee (1959), Bajaj Committee (1985) and High Power Committee (1987) were appointed in the past to suggest an organised health services and the community development programme where nurse would be an active mediator to attain the goal. But even almost half a century after independence, our nursing education and service are modelled on the same British pattern. Our heritage of nursing education in Orissa as well as in India has been "more academic than pragmatic, more global or international than national, more hospital than community oriented, more episodic than total management and a more individual than a group concern". Consequently, the nursing professionals in our country or state lack a pragmatic approach to the problem of educational change to suit the national health needs.

An examination of the reports and findings of several committees formed at the national level will serve a useful purpose. Of course, no such Committee has been formed so far to evaluate the socio–economic status of nurses in Orissa.

Bhore Committee (1946)

The conditions in which nurses have hitherto been required to carry on their profession in this country are recognised by all thinking persons to be deplorable. So long as such conditions would continue to prevail, Indian women from more educated and respectable families would hesitate to come to this profession in appreciable number.

The committee summarised the lacunae in the service conditions of nurses under five heads. These are (1) Lack of professional status any (2) Underpaid senior positions, (3) Grossly understaffed hospitals with consequent over work, (4) Deplorable living conditions with gross overcrowding, (5) Imbalanced diet, and (6) Absence of pension scheme.

The proposed remedies prescribed by the Committee were (1) Granting of gazetted rank to person on the basis of salary, (2) Revision of salaries to make the profession attractive, (3) Attempt to reach the International Standard of one nurse to three beds, (4) Fresh and vigorous approach to the problem of accommodation and diet, and (5) Inauguration of the pension and provident fund scheme.

2. As regards training facilities the Committee's proposals include the establishment of preliminary training schools for midwives, public health nurses and hospital social workers.
3. The Committee also suggested for two grades in nursing profession (a junior grade and a senior grade) training facilities. The entrance qualification for the former was recommended to be a complete course of matriculation.
4. Further, the Committee recommended the establishment of nursing colleges in order to provide a five year degree course in nursing as well as advanced courses in hospital nursing administration in the teaching of nurses and training of public health supervisors.
5. Owing to the existing social conditions and customs in certain parts of India, male nurses will have to play an important role in the health programme. So they should be trained and employed in large numbers in the male

wards and male outpatient departments of public hospitals, thus releasing women workers for other work.

6. The committee made some specific proposals in regard to the training of public health nurses. Their stress was given on preventive education and integration of class room instruction in arts/science/social studies with the work experience in hospital, house keeping and community services.

7. Existing training schools for midwives require considerable improvement. The most serious drawbacks are (i) lack of properly trained and well equipped supervisory staff; (ii) lack of facilities for antenatal and postnatal work; (iii) lack of domiciliary practice; and (iv) lack of opportunities for witnessing complicated cases of labour. It has laid down certain requirement which should be met before an institution is recognised as a training centre for midwives and also made detailed recommendations for their training courses.

8. Regulation of the Nursing Profession, including those of Midwives and Health Visitors.

   (i) At present the regulation of the nursing profession which includes those of midwives and health visitors, is vested in Provincial Nursing Councils which maintain registers of persons who have completed approved courses of training in institutions recognised by them for the purpose and have passed the prescribed examinations. Persons so registered are entitled to practice the profession in their won province. Arrangements for reciprocity with other provinces exist to a degree which varies with the nursing councils concerned.

   (ii) It recommended the creation of an All India Nursing Council to co–ordinate the activities of the provincial councils, to lay down minimum educational standards and to safeguard their maintenance. Questions of reciprocity within and outside India should be the concern of this Central Nursing Council. It recommended the maintenance of an All

India Register by this Council, with separate schedules for the entry of approved qualifications in general nursing, higher nursing, public health nursing, midwifery and health visiting.

(iii) The power to take disciplinary action should continue in the first instance, to be vested, as at present, in the Provincial Councils, but there should be a right of appeal to All India Nursing Council over their decisions, with additional provision for further appeal to the Federal Court in circumstances similar to those that prevails in the United Kingdom, where an appeal lies to the High Court against the decision of General Nursing Council.

Shetty Committee (1953)

The Committee has made the following recommendations on nursing training:

1. Recruitment of additional staff and the necessary staff for supervision and teaching, in the existing centres as a first step towards increasing the number of nursing personnel.
2. Creation of nursing staff posts in the institutions and in the public health field to absorb the additional number of trained nurses.
3. Appointment of auxiliary nurses and midwives to supplement service in wards which are not used to train nurses. Establishment of training centres in District Headquarters hospitals for auxiliary nurses and midwives.
4. Improvement in conditions of training of nurses giving priority to:
   (a) provisions of adequate living accommodation;
   (b) proper facilities for practical work and adequate training for sister tutors and ward sisters;
   (c) proper care of students health;
   (d) raising of educational standards wherever possible and
   (e) short working hours.

5. Better publicity to the potentialities of nursing as a career.
6. Special consideration to personality and home background when recruiting students, provided that they meet other minimum requirements and constitution of Selection Committee comprising the medical and Nursing Superintendents and Sister Tutor.
7. Ordinarily, married women, unless widowed or separated from their husbands, not to be admitted for training. Students not to be allowed to marry during training period.
8. Minimum requirements for admission to training schools to be in accordance with the regulations of the Indian Nursing Council.
9. Medium of instruction to be decided by each state. Individual training centres should also have discretion to decide this question.
10. Setting up a system of counseling of students and experienced sister belong assigned to a group of students for this purpose.
11. Compulsory residential training.
12. Adequate provision of stipend and allowance to meet messing, uniform and laundry expenses.
13. Execution of a 2 year bond by the student trainees.
14. Proportional recruitment to men and student nurses keeping in view the employment opportunities.

The recommendations on nursing services pertain to the following:

1. Appointment of Superintendent of Nursing Services in each state.
2. Combining the nursing service for hospitals and that for the public health field into one service. Inclusion of experience of public health and domiciliary nursing in the basic course for nurses and midwives.

Mudaliar Committee (1959–61)

The Mudaliar Committee made the following recommendations:

1. There should be three grades of nurses, viz. the basic nurse with four years of training, the auxiliary nurse midwives with two years of training and the nurse with a degree qualification.
2. Candidates admitted to the general nursing course should have the minimum qualification of matriculation or its equivalent, and candidates for the degree course should have passed the higher secondary or pre–university examination.
3. In view of the need for securing a large number of recruits for the nursing profession the age of admission may be relaxed to sixteen (16) in suitable cases as a transitional measure particularly in States where there are difficulties in recruiting candidates at the age of 17.
4. The medium of instruction should preferably be English for the general nursing course, while the degree course should be taught only in English.
5. Nurse pupils should not be over–burdened with the routine duties in hospitals, but more attention should be given to training and practical experience. They should not be subjected to too many spells of night duty in hospitals.
6. A large number of hospitals in the country can be utilised for Nursing Schools. District headquarters hospitals with a bed strength of 75 to 100 should also be utilised for this purpose.
7. The minimum number of admissions to be course should be 12.
8. Student nurses should be provided with free furnished accommodation in hospitals, free board, free supply of uniforms, laundry arrangements, free books, free medical services, medical check up twice a year and suitable recreational facilities. The stipend during training should be a minimum of Rs.35 with an increase of Rs.10 every year.
9. There should be a Nursing Advisory Committee in each school for advising on admissions and welfare of the trainees.

10. Each nursing school have its own budget.
11. The training of auxiliary nurse midwives should be continued and extended, because it will be necessary for a longtime to come to have a second line of trained personnel to meet the need of the country.
12. The number of auxiliary nurse midwives to be trained should be phased at in such way that there will be one auxiliary nurse midwife for 5,000 population.
13. Time has come to give a fresh look to the type to training imparted at present to health visitors. A public health nurse with a basic nursing qualification and one year's further training particularly in domiciliary care and other public health aspects of community work would be more suitable in this present context.
14. Any person trained in one category of nursing should get an opportunity of being trained in the next higher grade under conditions to be specified by the Indian Nursing Council.
15. Provision of higher training for the general sick nurse, public health nurse, paediatric nurse, mental nurse, theatre nurse, sister tutor and nursing administrator.
16. Promotion of degree course nurses or basic nurses to the post of higher responsibility be considered only after a minimum of three to five years of practical experience after obtaining the minimum qualification.
17. Male nurses be trained only for certain type of work like work in the mental hospitals, army hospitals, VD clinics and rehabilitation centres.
18. Fairly pleasant terms of service to attract to the nursing profession and to lure them away from clerical jobs.

The suggestions and recommendations made by different committee set up by government of India from time to time have not actually been accepted and operated in all the States. The appointment of High Power Committee on 25th August, 1987 by the Government of India to review the conditions of services, status and allied problems of the nursing profession has, therefore, come as a very pleasant development in this line. The Committee was headed by Dr. (Mrs) Jyoti Trivedi, formerly Vice–Chancellor of SNDT University for women, Bombay. It had 11 other members including the President of TNAI Mr CPB Kurup and Mrs. M. Chabook, President, Indian Nursing Council and a former President of TNAI.

The terms of reference of the Committee are as follows.

(i) To look into the existing working conditions of nurses with particular reference to status of the Nursing care services, both in rural and urban areas.

(ii) To study and recommend the staffing norms necessary for providing adequate nursing personnel required to give the best possible care, both in the hospitals and community.

(iii) To look into the training of all categories and levels of nursing and midwifery personnel to meet the nursing manpower needs at all levels of health services and education.

(iv) To study and clarify the role of nursing personnel in the health care delivery system including their interaction with other members of the Health team at every level of health services management.

(v) To examine the need for organisation of the nursing services at the National, State, District and lower levels with particular references to the need for planning and implementation of comprehensive nursing care services with the overall health care system of the country at the respective levels.

(vi) To look into all other aspects which the committee may consider relevant with reference to their terms of reference, and

(vii) While considering the various issues under the above terms of reference, the committee will hold consultation with the state government.

Though all India Committees have been constituted from time to time to study and review the status and working conditions of the nursing profession, the government of Orissa has never made any attempt to evaluate the working and living conditions of the nurses at the State level.

The High Power Committee made recommendations on the working conditions, education and condition of services of the nursing personnel. It emphasises on bringing at uniformity in the employment procedure, job description of all categories of nurses, reduction of working hours and work load, improvement of working facilities, uniformity of pay and allowances, extension of promotional opportunities, provision of career development, accommodation and transport facilities, provision of special incentives, protection from occupational hazards and provision of additional facilities to nurses working in the rural areas.

Similarly, in the field of education, they recommended the upgradation of nursing schools of medical college hospitals to degree level and expansion of B.Sc. Nursing degree and postgraduate and provision of central assistance to nursing education. Recommendations were also made on clear–cut policies relating the nursing services, staffing of the hospitals, relief of nurses from non–nursing duties, improvement of patients' care and giving gazetted rank to the nursing sister etc. The High Power Committee also recommended to raise the position and status of nursing personnel working in the Directorates and to enable nurses to participate in policy making and decision making. They recommended the setting up of Nursing Advisory Committee/ Board to advise the government on nursing issues.

The Aftermath of National Level Committees

A college of nursing was established in 1946 at New Delhi with affiliation to the University of Delhi to offer a 4 year B.Sc. (Hons.) degree in Nursing. Training of male nurses was continued and two grades of Nursing courses–Senior 'A' Grade and Junior 'B' Grade–were started. Secondly, on the recommendation of Bhore Committee the Indian Nursing Council was established in 1947 to regulate the standards of nursing education. In the year 1950, the Indian Nursing Council took the following three important decision.

1. Retention of only two standards of training for nursing and midwifery–(a) A full course in nursing of 3 years duration followed by a course in midwifery of a minimum period of six months, and (b) A course of Auxiliary Nurse–Midwife for 2 years.

2. The minimum educational requirements for entrance to the Nursing course to be matriculation and for auxiliary nurse midwifery the educational standards were kept at 7th or 8th class period.
3. The Auxiliary Nurse–Midwifery course to replace the various courses for the junior grade certificates and the course in midwifery for candidates other than nurses.

Thirdly, new schools at district level for training of auxiliary nurse–midwives and training of nurses were opened. Selection Committees were formed for selection of student nurses. Public Health Nursing was integrated in General Nursing and Midwifery Course to enable the qualified nurses to work either in hospitals or community. Fourthly, on the recommendation of Mudaliar Committee (1959–61), three grades of training of nurses were further strengthened–*i.e.,* (a) B.Sc. degree (4 years), (b) General Nursing and Midwifery (3½ years), and (c) Auxiliary nursing training of 2 years. Qualifications recommended for admission to three grades of training programme were implemented. The Public Health Nursing Course of 10 months duration was started for qualified nurses to prepare Public Health Nurses instead of Lady Health Visitors. Nurses holding degree in Nursing were considered for higher posts only after minimum 2–3 years of practical experience. Master's degree in Nursing was started in 1959 for providing opportunities for B.Sc. degree holders. Efforts were made to increase stipend and living conditions of student nurses. Courses in Psychiatric Nursing and paediatric Nursing were initiated.

Committees and their Impacts in Orissa

Being one of the States in the Indian Union, the rules and regulations in vogue at the national level are bound to influence directly and indirectly the working and operations of nursing services in Orissa. The Board of nursing education in Orissa, a body at par with the Indian Nursing Council at the State level, had laid down a three and half year course for the nursing students on 25th October, 1981. In the first year, there were three theory papers and one practical paper in Fundamental Nursing. In the second year there were three theory and one practical paper in Advanced Nursing and in the third year there were only three practical papers. The last six months was devoted to a midwifery course in which teaching was based on Gynaecology and Obstetrics. But the new syllabus introduced in 1989 is having three theory papers and one practical paper in the first year, three practical papers in the second year and only one paper in Midwifery in the third year.

Even though the Indian Nursing Council (INC) approved regulations under section 16(1)(g) of the INC Act, 1947 for Post–Graduate teaching in six special fields, such as (i) medical Surgical Nursing, (ii) Paediatric Nursing (Child Health), (iii) Midwifery (Obstetrics), (iv) Community Health Nursing, (v) Maternal Child Health Nursing, (vi) Psychiatric Nursing, it is yet to be introduced. The duration of the Post–Graduate Course is for two years or four semesters. The maximum number of students to be admitted in a year is two only. But Orissa does not have a Post–Graduate institution. There is only B.Sc. Nursing college at Berhampur in Ganjam District.

Training of nurses is primarily a State subject. The entrance requirements diploma/certificate course in Nursing have been raised by the Centre. Since 1981 from Matriculation to 12th class pass and it was given effect to State in 1989. This would enable the students to pursue higher studies in nursing at the University level. Selection of candidates for 240 seats in three medical college hospitals of Orissa is made purely on merit basis. In spite of appointments of several committees and their recommendations no spectacular steps have been taken to uplift the socio–economic status of nurses in society. Several changes in their pattern of education, training, administration and delegation of authority are necessary. Incentives in several forms are also needed to generate an urge in them to serve the society.

5.2 Prospects

The picture of nursing at the threshold of 21st century seems bleak unless a big thrust is given to it by right thinking citizens, government and nurses themselves. Nurses must be sensitive to the challenge and become more communicative to public and their medical colleagues through their actions and verbal communication. There is the need of a revolutionary change in the sphere of education, working conditions, living conditions and nursing practices. Further, their problems can be solved by computerisation, autonomy and participation in nursing administration.

5.2.1 Education and Training

Education and training hold the key to any progress. Though a handful of sample nurses affirm that their education and training are best suited to their work, the fact remains that there is a wide gap between the theory and practice. The real education and training they acquire is in the field, during their course of interaction with the patients. The following few measures would help improving the standard of education and training to a considerable extent.

(1) Laws and regulations should prescribe the basic requirements regarding nursing education and training and should empower the competent authority to supervise such education and training.

(2) There should be two levels of approved basic education and training: (a) an advanced level, designed to train professional nurses, sufficiently wide skill to enable them to serve at any complex unit, and (b) a less advanced level, designed to train ancillary nurses to enable them to work at less complex unit which require less skills and aptitude.

(3) There should be programmes of higher nursing education to prepare nursing personnel for the highest responsibilities in direct and supportive nursing care, in the administration of nursing services, in nursing education and in research and development.

(4) After three or five years, a nurse must attend a refresher course to keep her knowledge up to date. The Government should organise refresher course in which experts, doctors and matrons should give lectures and demonstration in new development and recent discoveries in medical science which are now introduced in educational stream and the disciplines.

(5) Nursing students should enjoy the rights and freedom like other students, subject only to limitation which are essential for their education and training.

(6) During their practical work, nursing students, should only be assigned tasks which correspond to their level

of preparation. Practical work should be carried out to serve their training needs rather than meeting their normal staff requirements.

(7) Nurses during their training period should receive precise knowledge about working conditions, and career prospects which will provide means for their economic, social and professional interests.

(8) Nursing personnel undergoing education and training abroad should be able to obtain appropriate financial aid on conditions to be determined by multi–lateral or bilateral agreements or national laws and regulations.

(9) When a nurse is appointed in a social department, she should get complete information about the nature of her job, her co–workers, supervisors, operating rules and procedure of work.

(10) A modern library with plenty of news letters, magazines, bulletins and current books of eminent authors should be available to all the nursing staff.

(11) There should be proportion between class–room teaching and work in wards. Simultaneously, there should be also correlation between theory taught in class–rooms and the practical in wards. A request may be made to the universities concerned to make suitable modifications in the admission rules.

(12) All General Nursing Diploma students passing out General Nursing Examination should put in one year's internship at the end of two years of which six months will be spent in the rural setting. Similarly, at the end of one and half year's Auxiliary Nurse Midwife Course, students shall have to put in six months of internship in the rural setting. For all the above courses, the relevant diplomas or degrees shall only be awarded after the candidate puts in two years' service in Government or in any other establishment in the State, unless she is selected for a specialised training.

(13) A specialised number of seats should be reserved for admission to medical colleges for the deserving

candidates who are diploma holders in nursing education and who have served in rural areas for at leas three years.

(14) Minimum age limit for both these Auxiliary Nurse Midwife and General Nursing Courses should be kept at sixteen years as on 31st December of the year of admission.

(15) One single factor than can be blamed for fall in standards of nursing education is the casual treatment of management of nursing schools. All requirements of standard of education, posts, curriculae, physical facilities laid down by the Orissa Nursing Council as well as Universities concerned, should be mandatory.

(16) College of Nursing imparting B.Sc. Nursing Courses in the Berhampur University should be fully upgraded as the Post Graduate institute of nursing education and two other B.Sc. Nursing courses be opened at Cuttack and Sambalpur to cater to the regional needs. Care should be taken to develop full–fledged teaching departments suitable for training degree courses of specialisation for nursing education.

(17) Selection of students for admission should be made purely on the basis of merit.

(18) Vocational guidance regarding nursing education should further strengthened through the Bureau of Technical Education as well as through mass media.

(19) Time–table for student nurses should be realistic and should not exceed eight hours per day. It should be properly divided between ward experience, laboratory and class–room training as laid down by Orissa Nursing Council.

(20) Adequate provision of residential hostel facilities for students.

(21) Organisation of appropriate refresher courses at selected nursing Schools.

(22) Semester system or block system of teaching in various subjects and conduction of examinations as adopted for

the medical course be introduced for nursing education as well.

(23) For the purpose of economy and optimisation of resources, all paramedical education should be pooled together with nursing as far as middle level of health team is concerned. After two years of basic training, the 3rd year should branch off into at least three main branches–Hospital Care, Community, Health Service and Laboratory Service. This measure may be useful in mitigating the deficiency of health personnel in the long–run as well as improve the quality of health services.

The present education imparts bookish knowledge where practical and clinical training is most inadequate. Theory taught in the class–room therefore, must be made more informative with the help of abundant use of audio–visual aids like transparencies, films, charts, models, video tapes etc. and the knowledge so gained need be well supported by practical bed–side training in wards or in outdoor visits. Education of nurses, therefore, should be stimulating rather than traditional. Laboratories for conducting practicals need be specious well ventilated with adequate number of fans, projectors, epidiascope and blackboards.

5.2.2 Working Problems and Solutions

Problems of long and abnormal duty hours, shortage of nursing personnel at peak hours of a day, non–nursing duties loaded over the nursing staff, responsibility for the breakage of hospital articles and the need for a neat and smart uniform should be attended to with imagination. Further both internal and external security in work place is also necessary.

The duty hours for all types of nurses are very long. During the day, they have to work for 7 to 10 hours and during the night, for 13 hours or even more. Compared to other offices these duty hours are certainly abnormally long and taxing. There is no fixed interval for rest which varies from about 15 minutes to one hour. Long and inconvenient duty hours are not matched by compensatory holiday for the nurses. Shortage of nursing staff is one of the reasons for the increase load of work on the existing staff. In three medical college hospitals, student nurses are engaged to compensate the shortage of staff but in rural areas where there are no nursing schools to supply student nurses to meet the shortage of hands, the existing staff has to work overtime. Further, the sanctioned number of beds in the hospitals are always ignored. To ensure better services to the patients admission need be made as per the accepted ration accepted by the Orissa Nursing Council.

The second problem to be tackled is the shortage of nursing hands at peak hours of the day in the medical college hospitals. From early morning till about lunch time, the nursing workload is, in fact, heavy. During afternoon and night hours it is lighter except for new admissions of patients in critical conditions. This situation results in split hours of duty from some nurses which is inconvenient for them. The solution to the problem of shortage of hands at peak hours of the day may be sought in employing nurses on part–time basis which will turn thousand of labour hours into productive services. This may solve the problem of unemployment to some extent and ultimately, the problem of hospital in regard to extra nursing hands.

Thirdly, one of the major problems of the staff nurses is non–nursing duties. The intensity of the problem increases due to absence of facilities like running water, medicines, surgical dressings, spirit, bandages, linen, cotton, bedsheets and towels in good numbers. The problem multiplies due to several other non–nursing duties of the existing staff like keeping registers of indent and issue of articles and records of drugs etc. which involve a lot of paper work and in the nature of a clerical job. Further, nurses are held responsible for existence and maintenance, repairs of machines and all sundry articles in the ward and for that they have to fill up number of forms, indents and registers everyday. It is very much time consuming and adds to the excess work burden. To reduce non–nursing work burden we may take the following steps.

(i) Development of a system of central store for supply of linen and sterile equipments,

(ii) A floor pharmacy system in medical college hospitals to solve the difficulty of indenting medicines and other supplies to avoid unnecessary procedural details of filling up indents etc.,

(iii) Department of a clerk to a number of wards to do the paper work,

(iv) Creation of a suitable managerial cadre like non–technical Administrative Deputy Superintendent to control staff and maintain deadstock registers of the hospitals,

(v) Breakage of articles to be regarded as joint responsibility of the entire staff rather than that of an individual one,

(vi) Confining the work of an efficient staff nurse to work like keeping health charts, medicine schedules accounts of drugs given to a particular patients and records of patient's admission and discharge etc. rather than assigning other nursing duties.

The fourth problem of a nurses is associated with a clean, neat and smart uniform. It is observed that a uniform gives a nurse an image of cleanliness discipline, alertness, devotion and kindness in society. Three sets of uniform should be supplied to each nurse per year through a centrally located garment unit to be established by the Government. Besides, the three medical college hospitals being largest hospitals in the State should provide facilities of getting the uniforms cleaned, starched and pressed free of cost at their laundry establishment.

Lastly, the greatest problem of nurses of work–place is security. Security is two dimensional, one is protective provisions of their health and another is associated with the security in night service from the hooligans and anti–social elements. To protect them from occupational hazards, they should be supplied with minimum medicines, adequate soaps, towels, well ventilated rest–rooms and nutritious foods in the hospital premises. Sometimes hospital premises are infested by anti–social elements at night which become unsafe for the nurse at night duty. Deployment of adequate security force is, therefore, necessary not only for the safety of nurses but also for the patients and their relatives. Measures if adopted in the lines suggested above would improve the working conditions of nurses to a considerable extent.

5.2.3 Living Conditions

A healthy living condition promotes a healthy physique and a healthy mind. Living conditions are associated with accommodation along with other modern amenities like free water supply and both rooms with good sanitary arrangements etc. The nature of the profession justifies provisions of accommodation within hospital campuses or in the vicinity of the hospitals. That would reduce the workload and late arrival and ensure safety and security at work place. The Government of Orissa has provided accommodation to 49 per cent of the nursing staff within the medical college hospital premises. If all the nurses could be provided with government accommodation, apart from the considerations stated above, there would be a perceptible increase in the overall efficiency.

Construction of quarters is expensive and it may not be possible on the part of the government to bear the burden so easily and instantaneously. To ease the situation, nurses may be provided with house building loans and advances and be encouraged to own their own houses in the area convenient to them. Besides, the government may provide messing allowance, ration allowance, washing allowance and uniform allowance etc. to increase their living standard and status in society. A healthy living atmosphere provides tremendous relief from terrible physical and mental strain.

5.2.4 Present Quality of Nursing Practice

Nursing service is gradually deteriorating and is completely turning to be mechanical. It has also deviated from professional ethics. If it continues to deteriorate at this rate, the entire profession may turn to be inhuman. Patients are the guests in the hospital and nurses are the hosts who look to their welfare. The duties of nurses are not only to assist doctors, but also they have to play an independent role in their areas with a kind, sympathetic and compassionate attitude. There is a saying that, **"God made mother because He could not be everywhere at all times".** This could be extended to the health system and we may say that it created a professional called a nurse (like a mother who is to be a female) because a doctor may not remain present everywhere at all times. But this noble profession has lost weight due to the following reasons.

(a) Haphazard planning of institutions without adequate physical facilities.

(b) Non–maintenance of ratio of nurses to patients and the consequential excess workload.

(c) Selection of candidates under pressure without giving due consideration for their will power and aptitude.

Any profession needs a sound base for qualitative practice in the field. Our future plan, therefore, should be as follows.

(i) Need based study, in service education and modern technical advanced training are required for this purpose.

(ii) Need based service or sterilization technique concerning patient's life and death is very much necessary.

(iii) Quarterly review meeting should be held with the state authority to find out practical shortcomings and solutions.

(iv) More emphasis should be given on practical training which is tremendously lacking.

(v) Involvement of Nursing personnel in planning is necessary to serve our purpose.

(vi) Selection for nursing of only those candidates who want to accept the profession with dedication.

To bring a qualitative improvement in nursing practice, expected change in administration and organisation should be made which may ensure professional dignity of nurses and nursing practice.

5.2.5 Computerisation

As the demand for improvement in the delivery of health care grows louder, the need for expanded and innovating training programme is necessary. This challenge of improved programme is met by way of Computer Aided Institution (CAI) and Computer Aided Education (CAE). Educational soft were consisting of teaching and training is now obsolete. Use of hardware technology like computer imparts training through a video screen, where the trainee remains in a physical contact with the computer system and ensure a more effective training. Teacher's capabilities and personal moods and attitudes are no longer a constraint. Class–room and clinical experiences, therefore, need by supplemented by CAI and CAE.

The three medical college hospitals are over crowded by patients in proportion to the nurses who would effectively meet the need. To add to this, there is voluminous amount of paper work to be handled. This leaves little time for patient care and chances of error increase due to manual computation, thereby making the system inefficient and inaccurate. However, with computerisation, they could resolve these problems.

In recent year, there has been a tremendous impetus towards computerisation in nursing. As the largest group of employees, the nurses are in a position to use computerisation technique significantly and derive benefits including (i) reduction of clerical work, (ii) reduction in printed forms, (iii) centralised patient care data, (iv) accurate accounts and information, (v) improved cost accounting (vi) possible reduction in length of patient's stay, (vii) dietary planning, and (viii) inventory control for drugs and other supplies.

Computerisation can be adopted, adapted and absorbed into virtually every area of nursing services. Computer can assist them in the following areas.

(a) Clinical Nursing,

(b) Nursing Administration,

(c) Nursing Education, and

(d) Nursing Research.

The process of Computerisation is explained in Fig. 18.

(a) Clinical Nursing

Computer plays an important part in nursing care, saves time and removes a considerable workload on nurses by taking over the routine documentation and other clerical functions such as records of treatment of books controlled drug book, investigation book, diet sheet, inventories of wards, medical and dispensary indent book and so on. These are time consuming activities which a nurse has to perform besides giving direct patient care. The time saved due to reduction in paper work allows the professionals to spend more time with the patient care such as feeding, sponging, meeting needs of the patients and providing psychological support to them.

Computer is equally more productive in monitoring the vital parameters in the care of patients who are critically ill (ECG, Systematic Arterial pressure, Pulmonary Arterial pressure, CVP, Heart Rate, B.P., Automated computer–assisted fluid and metabolic

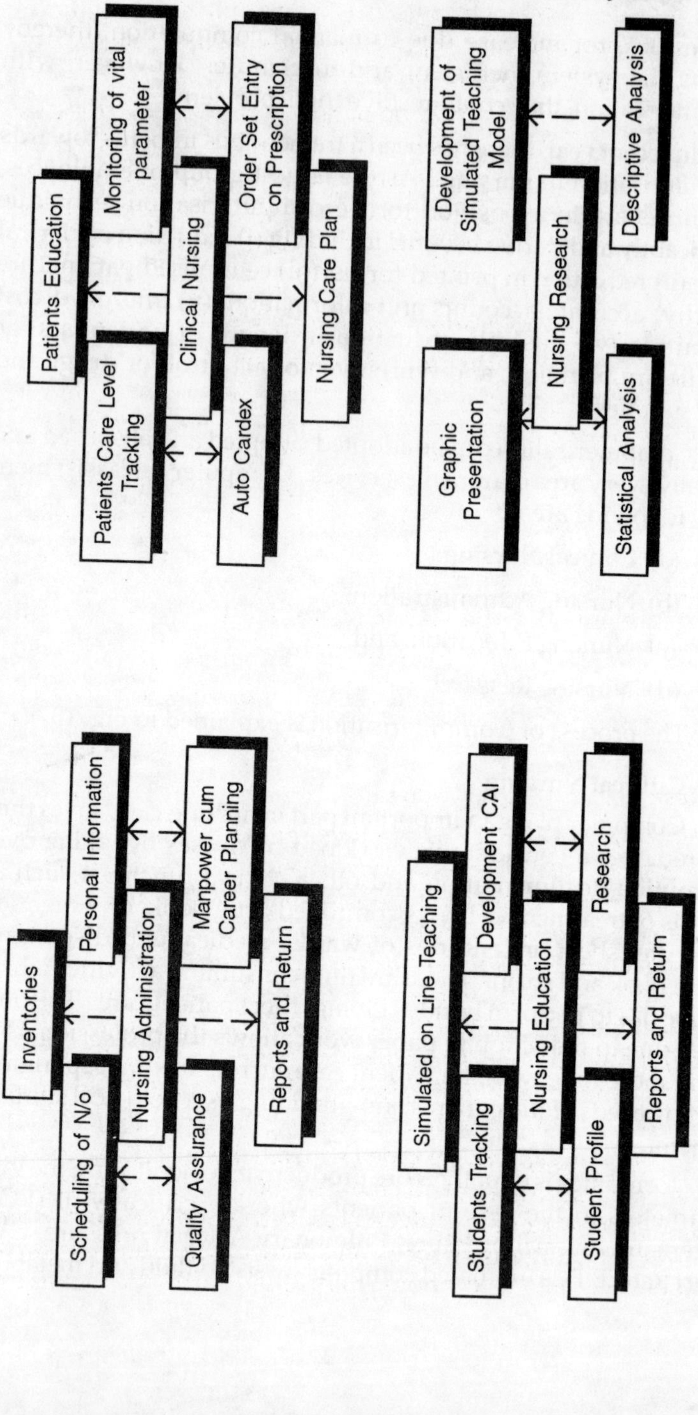

Fig. 18: Computerised Process

balance and TPR) and such a system could be built in the computer to alarm the nurses when parameter lies below the safe/normal range to take appropriate action in time.

Information entered in computer regarding patient care is not lost and easily available to physician and nurses through the use of remotely located terminals thus, helping in maintaining the continuity of patient care. Use of telephone is also minimised as the laboratory investigation values or reports are entered directly into the computer if the local areas net work is used.

(b) Nursing Administration

Because of its high speed processing and error–free transmission of data, computer can improve upon many routine functions of nursing service administration system by identifying those management tools that will improve efficiency while reducing cost and errors besides maintaining quality and effectiveness. The application of computer technology in nursing administration activities helps in assessing the patient needs and translating these needs into staffing requirements and policy–making, estimating workload, maintaining personnel record, medical record, career development, promotions and superannuation and resettlement. All these information which are prepared manually for every promotion board, selection for deputation courses and specialist training can easily be retrieved once computer is introduced.

(c) Research and Development

With the availability of highly sophisticated and versatile graphic system, both in terms of software and hardware, the design and development process has found a facility. **"Computer–Aided–Design"**, which was unheard of a few years ago. Such developments of a computer simulation to evaluate the clinical performance, a large cluster of data processing applications that directly or indirectly support basic and clinical nursing research, complex statistical analysis and colour graphic system are like dream tools for research in nursing. It removes inaccuracies from mathematical calculations thus, providing accuracy of statistics. Years of work can now be performed with relative ease, compressed into a few days or weeks with the help of this advancement in computer technology. Computer Aided Instruction and Computer Aided Education (CAI & CAE) is yet another major development in the field of computer technology. Through hardware means or

Computer Aided Instruction and Computer Aided Education (CAI & CAE), nursing conditions and workload problem could be solved to some extent.

5.2.6 Effective Organisations

Problems relating to nursing services and nursing education could be solved through effective organisation and administration. Nursing services are an important part of health team of the State and constitute an organisation. Such a large organisation could function effectively only if it has the following sound qualities.

(i) Unity of objective,

(ii) Specialisation: precise divisions of work,

(iii) Co–ordination of all efforts towards the common goal,

(iv) Clean unbroken line of authority,

(v) Authority equal to responsibility,

(vi) Efficiency: attainment of objectives with lowest possible cost,

(vii) Effective delegation,

(viii) Unity of Command,

(ix) Span of Control: limited number of sub–ordinates to each superior,

(x) Balance: in the size of various departments, between standardisation of procedures and flexibility, between centralisation and decentralisation, between span of control and chain of command,

(xi) Appropriate communication,

(xii) Optimum use of human resources, full scope of personal ability,

(xiii) Exception principle recurring decisions handled by lower level of managers in a routine manner and problems involving unusual matters referred to higher level,

(xiv) Flexibility of changing circumstances,

(xv) Systematic grouping of activities: departmentation,

(xvi) Definiteness: each activity contributing to the basic goals of the organisation with minimum of effort and maximum of efficiency on the part of the employee, and

(xvii) Scaler Principle: The degree of sincerity, responsibility and corresponding authority decreasing in relation to the levels of organisation structure from relatively complete responsibility and authority at the top to relatively little responsibility and authority at the lowest level–authority following downwards from the top of bottom–responsibility and accountability flowing upwards from the bottom to the top.

A large organisation like nursing services cannot be managed satisfactorily by overlapping or delegated responsibility. This is precisely what has happened to nursing services. Another defect in the present day administration of nurses is that it is rather loosely woven with multiple points of control such as the Office of the Director of medical Education and Research, Office or Director of Health Services, Matrons, Deputy Director of Nursing, medical Superintendents, District Health Officers and Public Health Nurses. This faculty of arrangement blocks the channels of communication. There is no clearcut definition of authority and responsibility of each office of management. There is no unity of command, decision making and balanced function over the nursing services. The entire machinery of administration of nursing services need be reorganised. There must be appropriate delegation of administrative and financial powers. Proper supervision, guidance and support must be given to nurses working throughout the organisation. Every member working in the organisation must have easy channel of approach without social, political and administrative difficulties to express her grievance and expect justice. To achieve the above objectives, the future nursing services could be administered on the following lines.

A nursing division (Fig. 19) need be established in which the highest managerial post would be that of the Chief Nursing Administrator; or still better, the post will be designated as a State Nurse. A Senior Nursing Personnel with necessary nursing qualifications and experience will hold the post of State Nurse. He or She should function in consultation with and under the guidance of the Director of Health Services and the Director of medical Education and Research, Orissa, in policy matters, planning, financial implications, matters of government commitment and advise the government in nursing matters. In fact, all such matters should be brought before a committee consisting of Director of Health Services, Director of medical Education and Research and the State Nurse for decision making. The Senior Director will be acting as Chairman and the State Nurse will be the Member Secretary of the Committee. The State Nurse will be responsible to both the Directors for co–ordinating activities of the nursing schools with that of the nursing services. There shall be two Deputy State Nurse to assist the State Nurse. One of them will be looking after the Nursing Education and the other one will take care of the Nursing Services. The state should be divided into three regions, with three Assistant State Nurse to head each region. The Assistant State Nurse should be in charge of both Nursing Education and

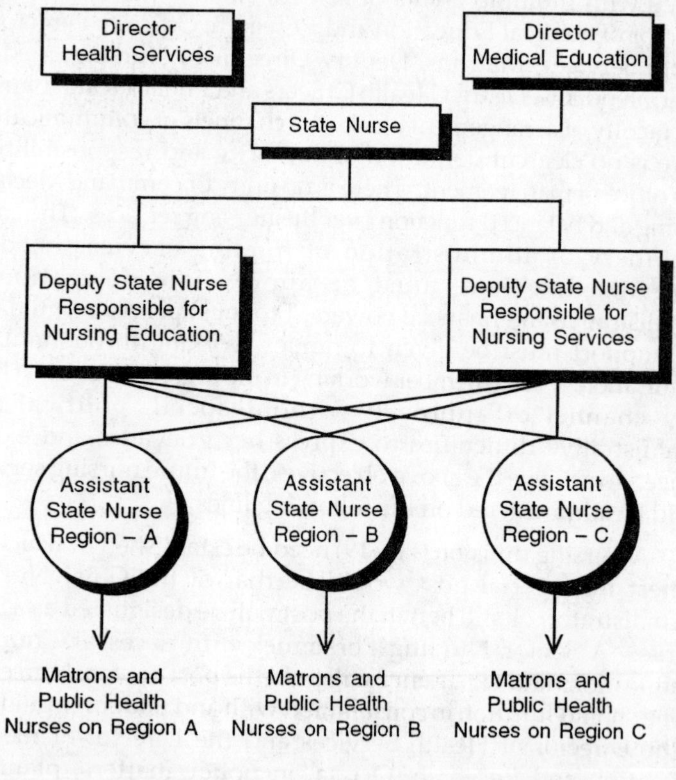

Fig. 19: Nursing Divisions explaining the Designations.

nursing services in the State. He or she will be the Regional Administrative Head of the nurses in the teaching and non–teaching institutions. The District Public Health Nurses and the Matrons of the hospitals in that region would work under the administrative control of the Regional Assistant State Nurse. It will determine the clear cut demarcation between responsibility and authority. This would mitigate the puzzle and confusion in the organisation to some extent. Once the organisation is established, all problems of nursing personnel could be solved that flow from bottom to the top through appropriate levels of management. As the chart reveals, the problems arising in regions A, B and C will be solved by Matrons and the District Public Health Nurses in their respective regions. Then they will be passed on to Assistant State Nurses of the concerned regions. The Assistant State Nurse will communicate with appropriate Deputy State Nurse and finally it will pass on to the State Nurse. For prompt and successful disposal of problems, it is absolutely necessary that duties and responsibilities of the various posts in the organisation are clearly defined and there is appropriate delegation of administrative and financial powers and control. For successful organisation and administration of Nursing Education and Nursing Services a structure of organisation on the lines of simple pyramidal plan of hierarchy should be built up and in this structure, the points of control and responsibility in decision making should be clearly stated. It is crystal clear that the structure and organisation in Bangladesh is comparatively a better one (Fig. 20). They have a separate Directorate of Nursing Services and there are several ranks of nursing officers with their clearcut power and limitation.

5.2.7 Professional Autonomy

Profession and autonomy are two sides of the same coin. In the national health scenario, equal to other health disciplines, nursing too is a powerful professional force. The profession is privileged to be called **"noble"**. But the same time the truth remains that nursing is a profession without autonomy. Autonomy in each dimension of nursing exists today in obscurity. Though nursing is a profession of paramount importance within the national health delivery system, yet it has been deliberately deprived of the autonomous status.

There have been parallel growth of many health disciplines. Out of these disciplines, medicine has emerged as the most dominant and unchallenged professional force and has secured a leading role, prescribing, dictating and shaping the course of events in nursing and thus, in the process curbing its own power by every inch. A new deal has been dotted out for nursing in the process, curtailing its authority to self–righteousness. The Post–Nightingale epoch of the professional growth has faltered. The harshest truth is that nursing today presents itself as a professional career of an illusory choice. With the administrative framework of the national health organisation, the status of nursing is obviously a source of embarrassment. There lie disorganisation and chaos in every aspect of nursing. Though nursing has a major

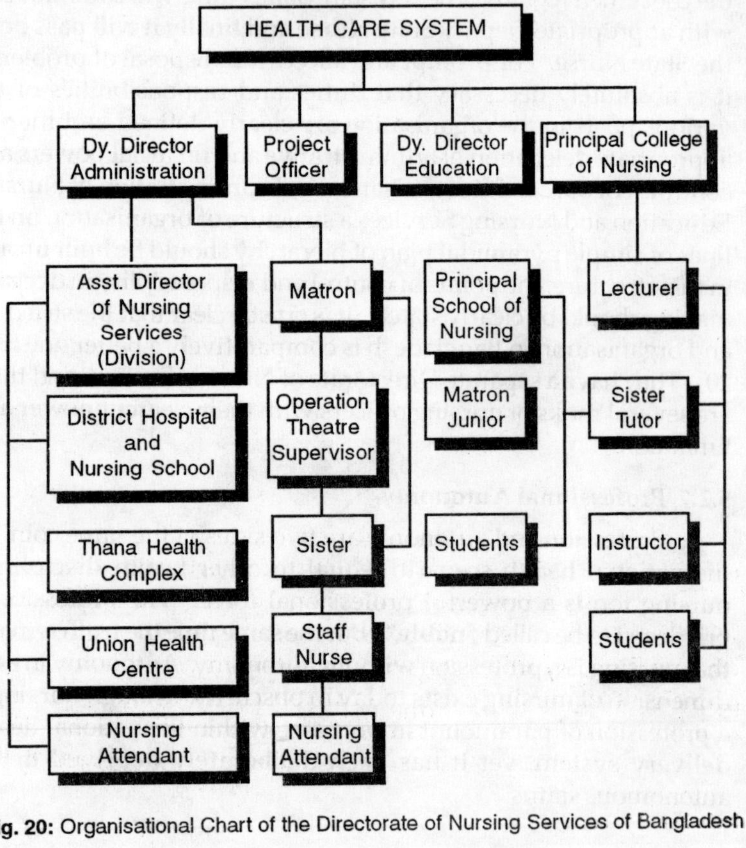

Fig. 20: Organisational Chart of the Directorate of Nursing Services of Bangladesh

role in executing health policies, it has very insignificant role in formulation of policies and strategies in three major professional areas such as nursing administration, major education and nursing services.

Though there has been enviable advancement in all dimensions of nursing, it is surprising to note that this situation remains unchanged and also unchallenged yet. There has been no awakening amongst the senior nurses to question the propriety of malpractices. The nurses occupying the administrative positions seem to be contented to remain merely a deputy or assistant to the Chief Policy–Maker, who is always a medical boss. Thus, the policies for nursing made by non–nurses remain deficient and defective. Within this repulsive atmosphere, nurse administrators are trained to function as common robots and carry out the faulty policies with her prescribed means within the restricted fields.

A great deal has happened in the advancements of nursing education too. But this tragic situation still exists in all nursing institutions. Appreciable progress of academic process in nursing has not been able to change its fate. Nursing long ago, left its status of vocation and climbed the steps of academic ladder to become a strong educational force. Nurses as educators with their proficiency and competence deserve comparisons with educators of other disciplines. But the nurse educators have restricted roles in exercising knowledge and competence, as the major portion of the nursing curriculum is covered by the medical teachers. This pattern exists from the elementary courses to specialised courses of nursing. The irony of this situation is that this pattern has prescribed by the nurses themselves. The system of evaluation in nursing is also not free from such endeavours. It is not a rare scene where medical teachers act as examiners and thus evaluators at all levels of nursing education. Thus, the critical analysis of the origin and evaluation of nursing unfolds some clues to today's status of nursing profession.

Early nursing in the world did not assume an autonomous stance. This was probably due to the fact that most nurses are women and the status of female was low. Nurses' functions were virtually trivialised and ignored. Nursing originated under the care of medical profession and thus, the growth was automatically moulded towards a subordinate position. As nursing took birth and grew under the protective hood of the medical authorities, medical profession accepted the legal guardianship of nursing. Medicine played a definite and concrete role in the modern nursing–there is no doubt about it. The nurses gratefully acknowledge the debt towards medical profession and recall with gratitude, the guidance, support and cooperation the profession received throughout. But it is an undeniable fact that this godfatherly attitude of medical profession has caused irreversible damage in the free growth of nursing as an independent profession. Nursing has not learnt to stand on its own feet. Nurses till today look forward to the medical authorities for guidance and direction. Nursing professionals after such a protective phase, lack courage to meet on their own today's demands and challenges. Lack of autonomy makes the professional activities sluggish and stagnant. Thus, gradually nursing gathered the dust and was looked down with a sort of contempt.

Nursing has been forced to remain within the medical compound and this has altered the course of nursing. The end result has been undesirable. Thus, over the year, nursing degraded from a noble profession to a parasitic occupation. Nurses seldom get an opportunity to give vent to their grievances. Any attempt by nurses to attain autonomy was prematurely and instantly aborted. The dragnet, the medical authority has spread and expanded and nurses become helpless to escape out of it.

On the other hand, lack of an earnest desire and initiative on the part of nurses of attain autonomy, is clearly evident. Majority of the nurses do not seem to resist actively their subordinate role. It will be an acid test to analyse the personality traits of many a nurse who can be pinned responsible for keeping themselves engaged in atrocious practices of assisting medical authorities to overpower the efforts of nurses to gain autonomy. These nurses possess inadequate academic preparation and are of little ability or competence in exercising their unflinching loyalty to the medical authorities have smoothly made their ascent to the professional superior roles. This has been possible because even till date the medical profession has a stake at all levels of selection of nurses.

Another problem of nursing is the loss of time in the long waiting the expectation that someday autonomy would come–but it did not. History reminds us that autonomy independence, freedom do not come, they are to be attained. There has been gradual growth of discontent amongst the younger nurses who are disillusioned by their own leaders and the medical counterparts. The professional reform is the main task today before the new generation of nurses. They are to resume the stir with renewed vigour to push it forward towards the path of autonomy. There can be no turning back. The demand is to be placed before the medical authorities. The slogan should be **"Let nurses be their own rulers".** The voice of the nurses should echo this feeling throughout till the power of autonomy is attained. The long cherished autonomy, if it can be achieved, will be a turning point for modern nursing. By making efforts to make themselves free from medical influence, nurses neither wish to be at war with their medical colleagues nor it would bring any split between two professions. This will probable be the end of a superior and subordinate relationship and a cordial kinship on mutual understanding and respect will begin.

Achieving autonomy alone will not solve all the problems of nursing. Sincere and earnest efforts need be made to preserve autonomy. Nurses are to be given opportunity to participate, not only in records, but also in reality, as members of interdisciplinary team in planning, programming, implementing and evaluating health and nursing services. For this purpose leaders are to be choosen from better brains, better intelligence and better preparations. Nurses are to assume leadership in all areas of functioning connected with nursing administration, nursing education and nursing services within the range of health service programme of the country. If other professions keep controlling nursing, it will never be able to develop its full potentials, if the voices of other professions override that of nursing the significant contribution made by nurses in the health services will be lost.

5.2.8 Essential Elements of a Developed Standard

The following elements are considered to be essential in developing the standard of the profession. (a) They should reflect the values, conditions and goals for advancement of the profession, (b) They are based on valid principles, (c) They are designed to help the profession to meet that changing health needs of the society, (d) They serve as a means for communicating the goals of nursing to the institutions, the state, the members of the profession, the public, (e) They include the broad range of practice dimensions in nursing.

The development of standards and related criterion measures is then guided by the basic principles which includes the general essential elements and addresses the specific essential elements according to specific functional area of nursing (Fig. 21). Standards of nursing practice focus on the individual practitioner and are, therefore, concerned with the role and function of the nurse. This role and function vary in different countries according to national development and health policies and according to the emerging degree of professionalism of the nurse and the numbers of varying levels of nursing personnel. Certain elements like nurse, nursing practice and nursing care should be considered as criterion measures. Essential elements for standards for Nursing Education are the education system, objectives of the programme, curriculum and nursing education resources and facilities.

It is the responsibility of the professional organisation to establish the standards for the profession in the form of definitions,

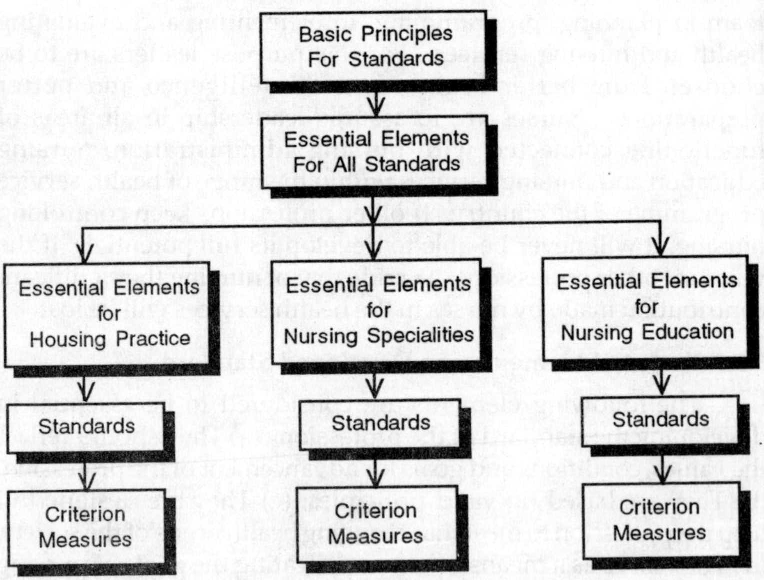

Fig. 21: Essential Elements for Development Standards.

ethical codes, education and service requirements and to communicate and promote these standards to the government and statutory authorities, the public, health and educational institutions and agencies and to the profession and its individual members. The process of developing nursing standards consists of three phases. These are

1. information and communication,
2. the development process, and
3. dissemination of standards.

In the initial phase, the task of Orissa Nursing Employees Association (ONEA) is to

— make decision to develop a provincial standards;
— allocate funds in the ONEA budget for the project;
— establish and select members of expert work group, and
— inform the Government/Ministry of Health and/or Chief Matron to develop standards for the profession and invite participation in process at various levels;
— widely circulate discussion paper to members and professional colleagues; and
— adopt and/or modify recommendations to workgroup.

In the second phase ONEA may establish a State Steering Committee for development and implementation of standards of oversee the carrying out of the plan of action and the recommendations of the discussion paper of the expert workgroup. The responsibility is to set up net work of state workgroups and taskforces, initiate consultation process with other health professions and ratify final version of standards. The third phase requires dissemination of standards to publish and circulate standards widely and institute a series of workshops through branches, work–group etc. to introduce the standards in appropriate workplaces and to develop more specific standards at the local level. The diagram illustrates the relationship of the various bodies involved in the development of State nursing standards and their major functions (Fig. 22).

5.2.9 A Solution

Forecasting future requirements is a difficult task due to the complexity of factors affecting demand and supply. In health, education and social service sectors, projections of requirement for manpower are often based on the concept **"needs"** and speak in terms consumer demand in a situation in which supply responds not to a market but to a political decision and the judgement of the government. For example, it might be felt that the availability of qualified doctors in every village is a desirable **"need"** but the question arises whether we have or do not have the capacity to pay for their services. It is, thus, necessary to make a distinction between the **"need"** that is the level of desirable social requirements of manpower and the **"effective demand"** which is based on economic considerations. For the better, the assessment or requirement should take into account not only the services which the society needs but also the capacity to pay for the services required.

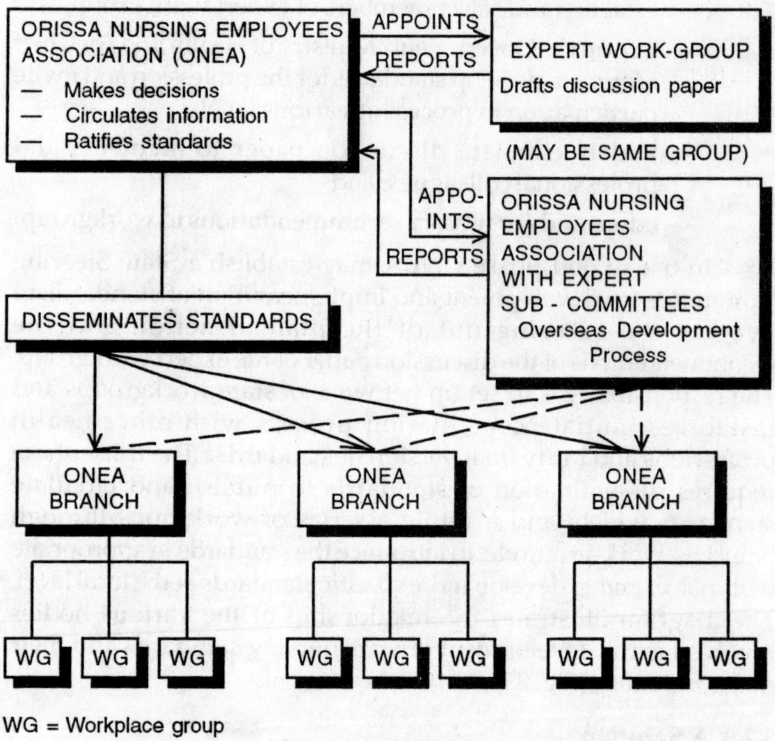

Fig. 22: Development process of state nursing standards.

It is necessary to make a distinction between **"Manpower requirements"** and **"Absorptive capacity".** Manpower requirements may be defined as minimum critical skill requirements by occupations. The assumption is that such skills are necessary, if not indispensable for the achievement of a programme of national development. Absorptive capacity is a term which refers to a country's capacity to provide some kind of useful employment for persons with some kind of useful qualification. In effect, the **"manpower requirements"** should express the minimum or essential needs; **"absorptive capacity"** should express the maximum number of persons who can be employed without encountering redundancy on serious underutilisation of skill. The concepts are very relevant in the present context of demand projections.

Demand used in a more restrictive or technical sense, refers to the amounts of the various types of health services that the population of a given area will seek and has the means to purchase at the prevailing prices with a given time period. From this demand the health manpower required to produce these services can be derived. Demand may also be used as a synonym for requirements. **"Need"** represents an estimation based on professional judgement in current medical technology of the number of workers or amount of services necessary to provide an optimum standard of health care. Need exceeds demand when there are insufficient resources to produce or purchase services in accordance with professionality determined needs.

The four methods of estimating the demand for health manpowers are health needs, service targets, health demand (or economic) and man power / population ratio. These four methods are presented as distinct entities though, in fact, each has a number of variants that overlap considerably with other methods. Broadly, the various approaches adopted for the choice of technique for projecting manpower demand could be classified as follows.

- — Normative Approach
- — Trend–Based Projections
- — ILOR–Trend Method (Incremental Labour Output Ratio)
- — Direct Enquiry Method
- — Component / Segment / Programmatic Approach

— Occupational–Industry Matrix Approach/Manpower Requirements Approach
— Rate of Return Approach
— Linear Programming/Econometric Models

Due to certain constraints of availability of data, generally four methods are used which are stated below.

1. Nurse–Doctor Ratio
2. Nurse–Population Ratio
3. Medical Services Users Approach and
4. Nurse–Bed Ratio.

The aggregative nurse–doctor ratio irrespective of their qualification gives a ratio of 0.8 nurses per doctor for the year 1986 while including the untrained nurse the ratio comes to 0.56 nurse per doctor. But the targets for achieving Nurse–Doctor Ratio in Public Health Services by the Government of India are 2.0 (1991) 2.5 (1996) and 3.0 (2001) (Fig. 23). Nurse–Population Ratio reveals that there were as many as 3,517 persons per nurse in 1986. Looking at the past trends, it has been assumed that the ratio will further improve to 3,000 in 1991, 2,500 in 1996 and 2,000 by the end of the century.

Medical Service User Approach takes into consideration the willingness and capacity of the people to pay for medical services. Demand in the economic sense is related to price and would generally be limited by financial resources of the family. Determining the amount to be incurred for medical services becomes a matter of allocating limited family income among alternative users. There is a relationship between family income and expenditure on health services. Demand for doctors can, therefore, be worked out on the basis of income elasticity of household expenditure on health services. On the basis of household data on consumer expenditure available from NSS rounds, the income elasticity of household expenditure on medical services has been assumed to be 1.5. This means that if per capita income goes by one per cent, households are inclined to increase their expenditure on health services by 0.5 per cent. Nurse Ratio has been used as a fairly common yardstick for estimating the requirements of nursing manpower. In this process the requirements of beds are first estimated keeping the growth of

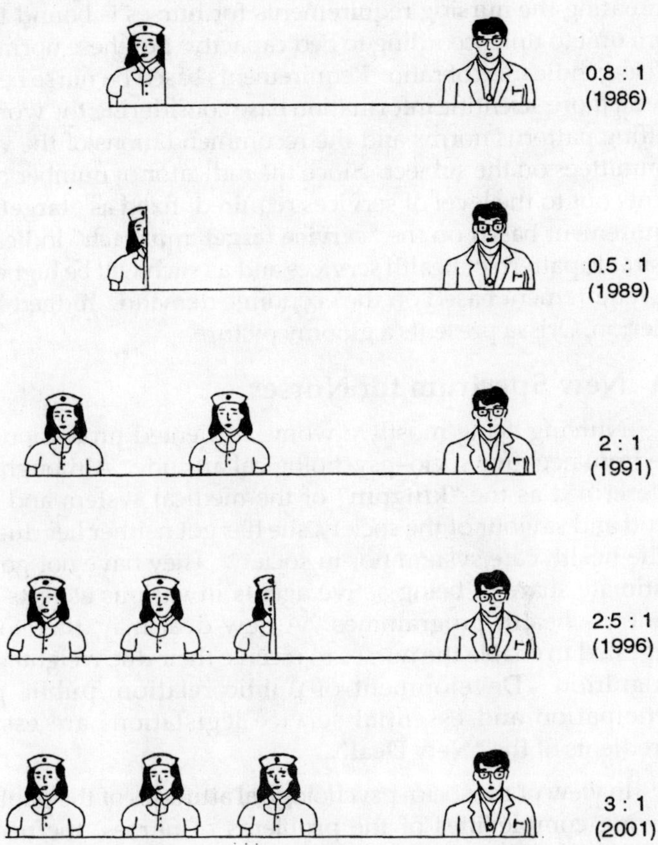

Fig. 23: Nurse – Doctor Ratio.

population in view and thereafter the requirements for nursing personnel are worked out.

The Bhore Committee suggested 20 to 30 beds for 10,000 population as a short–term plan and 50 to 60 beds as a long–term plan to be achieved by 1960. The Mudaliar Committee, however, suggested 10 beds per 10,000 population to be achieved in a period of 15 years. The current situation reveals that the bed population ratio has gradually improved and has come to 7 beds for every

10,000 population for the year AD 2000. Further, the question of estimating the nursing requirements for nurses is bound to vary from unit to unit according to bed capacity. But these norms have no clear indication of ratio. Requirements based on nurse bed ratio have a more scientific information base considering the workload, staffing patterns norms and the recommendations of the various committees on the subject. Since the indicator of number of beds points out to the level of services required, fixed as **"targets"**, the requirement based on the **"service target approach"** indicate the desirable pattern of health services and as such will be higher than the requirement based on the economic demand. Judged by any criterion, Orissa presents a gloomy picture.

5.3 New Spectrum for Nurses

Nursing being mostly a women–oriented profession is not free from negative socio–psychological attitude. Although nurse is described as the **"kingpin"** of the medical system and as the friend and saviour of the society, she has got neither her due place in the health care system nor in society. They have not got their legitimate share of being active agents in various aspects of the country's health programmes. A new deal may, therefore, be suggested to enable the nurses to receive their due weightage and recognition. Development of public relation, public policy participation and essential service legislations are essential ingredients of the **"New Deal"**.

In view of the socio–psychological attitudes of the public and growing complexities of the problems of nurses, the need for creating awareness among the members of the Government and public seems to be pertinent and urgent. Public relations practice is defined as the deliberate, planned and sustained effort to establish and maintain mutual understanding between an organisation and its public. A public relations unit of the nursing community may be created to sort out the internal problems of the nurses and to create forums to get them discussed and communicated to the appropriate authorities besides making constant efforts to build good image of the profession in the minds of the general public. Creation of public relations does not mean stagnation in the profession or shrinking in the responsibility. Frequent seminars, workshops, meetings, symposia, colloqua and conferences of this kind are to be arranged and the deliberations and proceedings be communicated to both the Government officials and the members of the public. Mass–media like local newspapers, radio and TV may be profitably utilised for communication. Special events like annual functions, cultural weeks, special awards, contests, meetings, visits of ministers of health and authorities etc. may be organised periodically. House journals in Oriya language may be edited for the internal circulation among the nurses. Their socio–cultural achievements should be publicised through mass–media to mobilise the public opinion.

The strength and value of any profession lies in its participation in public policies. Education is a vital force to adopt new skills to overcome new challenges. The nursing leaders should work hand in hand and create public awareness to participate in policy making. For increasing the effectiveness in participation, nurses should develop the following:

1. Know the system,
2. Identify the problem to work on,
3. Set clear goals and analysis,
4. Develop a plan of action,
5. Collect data,
6. Present to appropriate groups,
7. Be prepared well in advance,
8. Prepare for success or failure and follow–up,
9. Keep members informed of plans, and
10. Identify future areas to be work done.

All these factors are interacting and intracting to each other for development of effective participation in public policy which may be represented Fig. 24. In some countries certain categories of personnel are legally bound by an **"essential service"** legislation enacted to protect the health and safety of the public. Included in this category are nurses, teachers, firemen, police personnel and other occupation that provide essential services. The more complex methods of arriving at essential nursing services is utilised by an active nurses' union, with decision based on the following policy statement. "All services provided by nurses are necessary to the health and well being of the people they serve. While some nursing services can be interrupted temporarily, other involve literally essential matters of life and death".

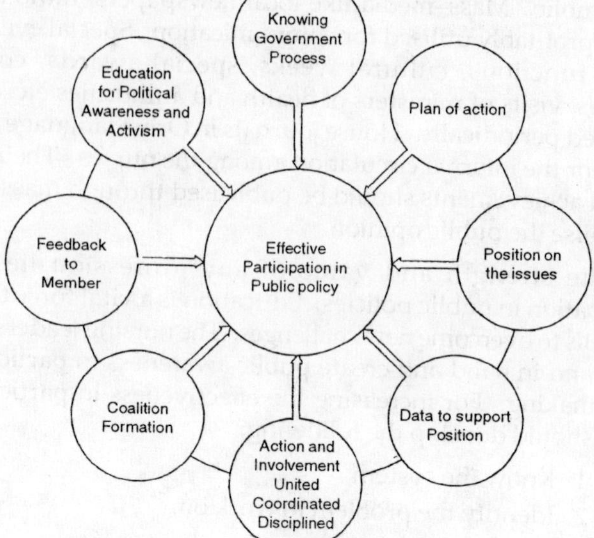

Fig. 24: Nursing participation in public policy.

Some of the objectives may be attained thorugh collective bargaining. The union is to decide how efficiently and effectively it could achieve the targets. But the criterion everywhere and always should be proper care of the patients. Law was a direct impact on the nurses, their workplace and the development of their practice. A basic understanding of the elements of the law will ficilitate the realisation of nurse's professional goals and the protection of their interests. Nurses' association must function within legal context. Using these complex infrastructure to its best advantage, they need to assist their members to improve the standards of health care in the coutnry as well as the professional, social and economic position of nurses.

Nursing personnel as well as workers should enjoy certain facilities in the sphere of working hours including regulations and compensation for overtime, convenient hours and shift work, weekly rest, paid annual holidays, educational leave, maternity leave and social security. But in the absence of proper organisational sturucture in the nursing services, lack of functional autonomy and exploitation, the socio–economic status of the nurses has not attained the height it deserves and a strong organisation can only restore the honour and diginity of the profession which has a glorious past and a colourful future.

Chapter 6

Summary and Conclusion

Nursing personnel, as front line health care providers, play a vital and crucial role in our national life. Recognising the potential contribution of nurses to primary health care; Dr. Halfdan Mahler, the former Director General of World Health Organisation, hailed nurses as the "**powerhouse of change**". Undoubtedly, nurses as such represent the greatest reservoir of undeveloped/underdeveloped leadership potential in the overall health care system in the country. This is a positive indication of the fact that they have the ability and strength to stand on an equal footing with other working men and women in many other fields of activity. However, the opportunities open to them are still few and far between India and Orissa. Judging from the angle of their contribution to society such a situation is unjust and undesirable. There are even today many social and economic constraints which restrict their active participation in their sphere of activities and inhibit articulation of their interests. This study was undertaken firstly, to assess the social status and dignity accorded to the nursing profession in the present day society, secondly, to evaluate their working conditions in the medical college hospitals of Orissa, thirdly, to measure their real economic benefits from their jobs and lastly, to evaluate the efficiency of policy measure of the Government of Orissa to uplift their socio–economic status.

The discussion on various issues relating to the life and work of nurses lead us to the conclusion that their problems are multidimensional and there is much to be desired in respect of improving their efficiency in the medical college hospitals. The social status of nurses in the project is measured by the parameters like social identity, marital status, educational status, domicile, religion, language and nature of the job. Nursing has no "**Identity**" as a medical profession. It is rather a para–medical profession. This nomenclature in respect of nursing personnel has long been dropped by WHO but it continues to appear in important documents like the Fourth Central Pay Commission Report (1986). Besides, the position of nurses in the labour market is governed by their state of education along with other factors like social taboos, cultural practices and employer's attitude. According to Lowies "**Primitive Society**" (1921), there are four determinants of the status of women, such as actual treatment, legal status, opportunity for social participation and extent of work. The determinants are independent units and the correlation among them is empirical rather than conceptual. The determinants in this study are nature of service, official accommodation, facilities in non–official accommodation, specialisation, educational status and marital status. Considering their nature of service, it is found that 93 (24.5 per cent) nurses are only permanent, 112 (29.6 per cent) nurses are temporary and 164 (45.91 per cent) are ignorant about their nature of service. As regards non–official accommodation 49.2 per cent have either no water supply or latrine. Lack of these facilities are only because of cheap accommodation. Regarding specialisation only 5.2 per cent are specialised in family planning, paediatrics and obstetrics. Specialisation is the most important factor to enhance the social status. There is definite correlation between occupational grade and degree of education received by occupants. Education is an important correlation and indicator of social status. From the educational point of view 61.2 per cent are M.E., 36.7 per cent are HSC, 1.8 per cent are +2 or I.A. and only 0.3 per cent are graduates. It clearly reveals that their low educational attainment has been a cause of their low social position. Judging from their marital status, it is noticed that nearly half of the nurses are unfortunate cases. They constitute widow (15 per cent), divorcee (2.5 per cent) and single cases (32 per cent) who have not attained the age of marriage. All those determinants in the study have established that nurses enjoy a low social status.

The study has also made an honest attempt to test the hypothesis that working conditions of nurses in three medical college hospitals of Orissa are satisfactory. There are the rules and regulations of International Labour Organisation pertaining to standard working conditions and working facilities and that provided to them in other States. The actual working conditions of nurses in medical college hospitals of Orissa have been compared with that of similar jobs elsewhere and international standards prescribed by International Labour Organisation. The stagnation and other accumulated problems in working conditions of nurses only go to prove that in the three medical college hospitals of Orissa their conditions are far from satisfactory.

(i) The study reveals the poor working conditions, lack of equipment and supplies, inappropriate nurse–patient ratio and dissatisfaction among nursing personnel. There are some basic factors that contribute to the deterioration in the quality care and give rise to many problems that indirectly affect the status of the nursing profession in the society adversely.

(ii) The workload of nurse continues to be heavy by any standards on account of

(a) unfavourable nurse–patient ratio which ranges from 1:10 to 1:30,

(b) admission of patients in excess of the bed capacity of wards,

(c) shortage of staff,

(d) inclusion of non–professional activities in their daily work and

(e) lack of sufficient equipment and supplies and time–consuming procedures to obtain even the bare minimum.

(iii) The study also reveals another problem that because of shortage of nursing personnel in hospitals, the community care apparatus and the educational institutions, the existing staff have to work for longer hours on broken shifts, abnormal shifts and even on public holidays. Such irregular working hours have an adverse impact on the personal life of nurses in as much as they have to isolate themselves from family functions, make frequent family and personal adjustments for abnormal hours of work. The current situation suggests that a Nursing Staff works longer than any other member of the working class. It ranges from 44 hours to 60 hours a week. The working hours need be reduced to 40 hours a week. Appropriate monetary compensation for overtime, evening and night shifts, public holidays and Sundays should be allowed to them just like Railways, Post and Telegraph and Industrial establishments.

(iv) Transport is a serious problem that frequently affects their working conditions. They have to commute during odd hours to distant places, make field trips and visit home and attend emergency calls and work during public strikes or "**Bundhs**".

(v) Another constituent of their working problem is lack of social security and special employment facilities. Social security schemes include provisions of financial compensation for working in risk areas, using protective devices, safe guarding nurses' rights and privileges in case of change of employment, temporary cessation of work and reentry into the profession. But nurses are deprived of the social security schemes to cover the entire medical expenditure, compensation for occupational health hazards and special consideration to nursing personnel as women employees.

(vi) The nursing profession with a majority of women employees involves considerable personal safety risks. But safety is not assured to our nurses. They run the risks from their employers, fellow workers, anti–social elements and outside visitors because they come in contact with the public while working and travelling during odd hours. Another point is that strenuous hours work expose nurses to undue mental and physical strain. Nursing personnel are exposed to additional health hazards like ionising radiation and anaesthic substances. The deplorable working conditions of nurses in three medical college hospitals of Orissa, therefore, negates the hypothesis of satisfactory working conditions.

An attempt has also been made to measure the economic status of nurses and to evaluate their economic benefits from the job.

(i) Remuneration is one of the important factors to study the economic status. It is seen that the prevailing remuneration is anomalous and discriminatory in many ways. Not to speak of the inherent constraints and service hazards, it is hardly commensurate with their qualifications, duties and responsibilities and experience. Their scale of pay is lower in comparison to similarly qualified incumbents in other allied professions like Junior Engineer and Army officials.

(ii) Lack of promotional opportunities is another determinant of low economic status. Two hundred forty seven (247) nurses completing 20 years of service have not tasted the first promotion in their life. The rest of the nurses (132 or 35 per cent) have got the promotional opportunity in name only. The posts of Chief Matron, Assistant Matron and Matron are day dream for them. Only 17.5 per cent nurses have an opportunity to be promoted as nursing sister after twenty five years of service. Further 3 (0.8) nurses have been promoted to the post of Assistant Matron and only one nurse (0.3) have got the rare opportunity of being the Matron in SCB Medical College hospital, Cuttack.

(iii) Landed property is taken as the third determinant of their economic status. It is found that 39 (10.3 per cent) nurses have lands varying from 0–5 acres placing them in the category of marginal farmers and none has more than 5 acres to boost up their economic status. Their other sources of income like private income and profits of investment are also marginal. Only one man has only a betel shop to supplement their income. 357 (94.2 per cent) nurses have General Provident Fund facility as a sort of compulsory saving and only 12 (3.2 per cent) nurses have post–office savings but none has any personal investment. They have no part–time income too although they work like machines during the duty hours and after.

(iv) Monetary benefit apart there is no real benefit for them. There is no free medical aid, travel and telephone facilities. They have to depend on the relatives or servants for child rearing. Nursing allowance and uniform allowance given to them are not at par with that of the centre or any other state like Karnataka and Maharasthtra. There is great disparity between uniform allowance, washing allowance, messing allowance, travelling and dearness allowance etc.

Thus, the hypothesis of adequate economic commensurate with their work and education is also negated.

Some of the committees at the national level point out the problems and prospects of nursing services. But no such committee has been appointed nor any policy has been made so far by the Government of Orissa to ensure appropriate socio–economic status to the nursing personnel. Career development opportunities in nursing are almost negligible and non–existent. Nearly 90 per cent of the nurses or more, stagnate in one position throughout their career and retire without getting a single promotion during the entire service. Such a situation is not only demoralising but also leads to aparthy among nurses affecting their effective functioning. The few higher posts available are, either vacant for years together or got abolished. Adoption of positive public policy is necessary to ensure their career development and provide a panacea to their long–standing problems. Since the Government is not seized of the problems of the nurses so far, the grievances multiply and give rise to widespread discontentment.

Conclusion

Nursing is both an art and a science. But these skills and knowledge of health preservation, practice and prevention of diseases should be applied outside the four walls of hospitals. Every profession is required to develop its own values to justify its existence. Nurses are accountable to patients who are actual consumers of their services, employers and fellow professionals. On the otherhand, the medical profession as a whole has came under severe criticism now a days. As the economic crisis becomes more and more pronounced, its manifestation may be seen easily in the health system also. But the people who see things differently from a very narrow angle, attribute many of the ills of the present day medical system to its malfunctioning, deterioration in nursing care and other such things.

From the foregoing analysis, it may be concluded that the socio–economic conditions of the nurses do not reflect a promising life pattern. Just like the weaker and exploited classes, they bear the major brunt of the burden of shortages, inflation and spiralling prices and the inadequacy and inefficiency of the administration. They have become the easiest targets, because they lack the power and appearance of cohesion and collective action. Besides that the efforts are not made for application of science and technology for evolving devices to reduce the drudgery of nurses in household work so as to enable them to enjoy some leisure after their busy hours in the hospitals. As long as these obstacles continue, the improvement of the status of nurses would remain a distant goal.

It is taken for granted that women join this nursing profession as a last resort. The services rendered by these qualified and trained nurses are also treated as manual services by the bosses as well as patients alike. It is again not a question of adequate monetary reward for which by and large individual nurse as well as the nursing community feel aggrieved. The informal discussion as well as their answers clearly the need of introducing other non–monetary incentives for them. Those include among other things even their psychological rehabilitation. Parameters in the study only confirm the multi–dimensional character of their problem. The social problem lies with their low social status. The very parameters or measuring rod to evaluate their social status are education, income martial status, nature of job, family set–up and nature of accommodation etc. All these parameters in the study clearly indicate the poor degree of social status accorded to the nurses in society. Effective measures need be adopted at individual and state level to enhance their educational, income, marital, job and family status.

Firstly, their role and importance in hospital, and their sense of devotion to duty may be given wide publicity through mass media like television, movies and radio to change the attitude of the public towards their job and services. Secondly, conditions need be created to attract qualified students to this job. Thirdly, by raising their income at par with such other categories of employees like junior engineers, their income status could be raised. Fourthly, without looking at their family set up and irrespective of caste and creed, their service and sacrifice may be judged as a criterion for enhancing social status.

Similarly, looking into realities of their living conditions, working conditions, income level and pay and perks, inference may be drawn that their economic benefit is not at par with their service and sacrifice towards society. Firstly, curative and preventive health care system may be developed to control unrestricted flow of patients to reduce their workload. Appointment of adequate number of staff, application of computer and clearcut demarcation of nature of work may reduce their work burden. In order to assess their economic benefit, the study has taken several measuring rods such as, service income, part–time income and private income as sources of income. Judging by their service income, it is revealed that it is one fourth of their real service rendered to society. The total time period required to attend the patients and to do other ancillary work is sufficiently longer than their assigned time. Secondly, they have no extra zeal for additional sources of income as their marginal sacrifice may not be compensated by higher marginal earning. Thirdly, they do not also spare time as is found on the Western Countries to earn something from private sources. Fourthly, their poor family background instead of helping in the enhancement of their economic status contributed in the deterioration of it in society.

In regard to the Government–policies and appointment of committees with a view to ensuring the upliftment of the nursing community, committees like Bhore Committee, Shetty Committee, Mudaliar Committee and High Power Committee appointed at the national level to suggest measures to socio–economic status of nurses, have never inspired the Government of Orissa to take appropriate steps in the right direction. Steps have not been taken to reduce their workload either by computerisation or by appointment of additional hands. In Orissa, recruitment to nursing posts by the State has been postponed since 1985. Students of five batches or so, therefore, remain unemployed. Ways and means need be devised to solve this problem. Measures also need be taken to enhance the socio–economic status of the nurses in the state after the issue is being evaluated by a high–power committee or a working group.

In Orissa, the very foundation of nursing structure need be strengthened. Firstly, nurse should have a strong base in the biological and social sciences to cater to the changing needs of society and science. Secondly, nursing administration in Orissa follows a hierarchical structure of management. Some amount of flexibility is necessary to reduce the amount of frustration of nurses in the state. A clear division of power and responsibility among all classes of nurses and medical team is necessary to avoid conflict or clash of interest in the medical team. In order to ensure coordination and greater functional efficiency of nursing services in the state, it is essential that all nursing personnel need be technically as well as administratively under the control of the nursing personnel themselves as per the suggested Fig. 21 for Orissa. It is important to consider nursing as a science based profession rather than a traditional, intuitive, task oriented and ritual practice. Perhaps the terms nursing sciences could be adopted for nursing community. In a State like Orissa as well as in a country like India where nursing is still not considered as a respectable profession, many young women are hesitant to come to this profession and perhaps the change of terminology may load to better social acceptance and marked improvement in the conditions and status of the nurses in the days ahead.

Bibliography

Abana, J. What a Public Health Nurse Is. *The Nursing Journal of India,* 1948, 2, 58.

Alber,t J. Reiss Jr. *Occupations and Social Status.* The Free Press, New York, Collier–Macmillan Ltd., London, 1977, 351.

Allen, L.A. *Management and Organisation.* International Student Series, McGraw–Hill Book Co. Inc., New York and Kogakusha Co. Ltd., Tokyo, 1958, 116.

Basu, M.N. *Work Measurement as a basis for calculating Nursing Establishment.* Leeds Regional hospital Board, 1979.

Bellows, R.M. *Psychology of Personnel in Business and Industry,* New York, Prentice–Hall, 1949, 288.

Berstein, E. *A study of Direct Nursing Care consumed by patients of varying Degree of Illness.* New York University, New York, 1968, 331.

Bhargav, S. Introspection : A Prerequisite for Emancipation. *Nursing Forum,* 1978, 3, 317.

Bhore Committee (The Health Survey and Development Committee) 1943–46.

Bopegamage, A. and Veeraraghaban, P.V. *Status Images in Changing India.* Australia and New Zealand Book Co. Pvt. Ltd., Thomas Street, Chatswood, NSW, 1977.

Cruz, J.V.D. and Bottorff, J.L. *A Multiple Assignment Model for Staffing Nursing Units, Operational Research Division.* John Hopkins Press, Baltimore, 1985.

Dablolkar, V.A. Life and Labour of Employed Women in Poona. Ph.D. Thesis. University of Poona, 1960.

Davis, K. *Organisational Behaviour at Work.* Fifth Edition, Tata McGraw Hill Publishing Co. Ltd., New Delhi, 1977, 13.

Gorwin, J.D. The Basic Training of the Public Health Nurse. *The Nursing Journal of India,* 1946, 4, 132.

Guion, R.M. Industrial Morale. The Problem of Terminology, *Personal Psychology.* 1958, 62.

Harner, P. and Lehma, H. *Nursing Education in India : Its relevance in Provision of Primary Health Care.* Wiley Eastern Ltd., New Delhi, 1983.

Harold, K. and Cyril, D. *Essentials of Management.* Second Edition, Tata McGraw–Hill Publishing Co. Ltd., New Delhi, 1978, 180.

High Power Committee on Nursing and Nursing Profession, 1988–89.

Kharpade, S. Nurses, Sheet Anchor of Health Care Delivery System. *The Nursing Journal of India,* 1988, LIX(12), 311.

Kind, E.M. A Conceptual framework of Reference for Nursing. *Nursing Research,* 1968, 17(1), 27.

Learned, P.E.; Ulrich, N.D. and Booz, R.D. *Executive Action and Division of Research.* Harvard University, Boston, 1951, 113.

Levine, M.D. and Philips, P.J. *Factors Affecting Staffing levels and Patterns of Nursing Education,* Washington, U.S. Government Printing Office, 1975.

Likert, R. and Willits, J.M. *Morale and Agency Management.* Hartford : Life Insurance Sales Research Bureau, 1941, 1, 27.

Lowie, R.H. *The Study of Man.* Persons Talcott, A revised analytical approach to the theory of social stratification, 1958.

Mathur, P.N. Medical Manpower Requirement and supply upto 2000 A.D. *Manpower Journal,* 1982, XVIII(3), 193.

Maslow, A.H. A Theory of Human Motivation. *Psychological Review,* 1943, 50, 396.

Maslow, A.H. *Motivation and Personality.* Harper and Row Publishers, New York, 1954.

Morgan, K.W. *The Religion of Hindus.* New York, 1953, 31.

Moore, W.E. *Management Process in Health Care.* Voluntary Health Association of India, New Delhi, 1978, 42.

Mudaliar Committee (The Health Survey and Planning Committee) 1959–61.

Nagpal, N. *Primary Health Care : Role of the Nurse in South Asian Perspective.* TNAI, New Delhi, 1984, 16.

Nagpal, N. Task before the High Power Committee of Nurses. *The Nursing Journal of India,* 1987, LXXVII(II), 283.

Newcomb, T.M. *Motivation in Social Behaviour.* In current theory and Research in Motivation, Lincon, University of Nebraska Press, 1953, 149.

Newcomb, T.M. The Prediction of Inter–personal Attraction. *American Psychology,* 1956, 11, 579.

Official Bulletin – International Labour Offices Conventions and Recommendations. Resolutions and Additional Texts and Decisions, 63rd International Labour Conference, Geneva, 1977, 1.

Park, J.E. and Park, K. *Text book of Preventive and Social Medicine.* 11th Ed., M/s. Banarasidas Bhanot, 1982, 32.

Park, K. *Management Process in Health Care.* Voluntary Health Association of India, New Delhi, 1982.

Phillips, J.R. Health Care Provides Relationship : A Matter of Reciprocity. *Nursing Outlook,* 1979, 27, 788.

Putnum, M.L. Improving Employee Relations. *Personnel J.,* 1930, 8, 325.

Rahudkar, W.B. The Arts, Science and Vocation in Evolution. *Contact*–59, 1980, 10.

Rao, M.S.A. Health Care in the context of Self Reliant Development. *Contact*–32, 1976, 13.

Report of Geneva Christian Medical Commission, 1974.

Report of World Health Forum, 1987.

Senior, O. *Dependency and Establishments.* Royal College of Nursing, United Kingdom, 1979.

Shivran, C., Rajana, M.S. and Vastard, A.B. *Work Measurement as a basis for calculating nursing establishment.* Leeds Regional Hospital Board, 1984.

Sherlekar, S.A. *Modern Business Organisation and Management : Systems Approach.* First Edition, Himalaya Publishing House, Bombay, 1978, 282.

Shetty Committee (Committee to review conditions of Service), 1954.

Smoke Nuisance Act, 1984.

Sood, R.K. Position paper in Nursing Education in India. *The Nursing Journal of India,* 1987, LXXVIII(4), 93.

Sood, R.K. Nursing services in India. *The Nursing Journal of India,* 1988, LXXIX(12), 318.

Timke, J. and Sweezy, A.M. *Time of Care.* Royal College of Nursing, United Kingdom, 1982, VIII(2), 328.

Townsend, R. *Up the Organisation.* Michael Joseph Ltd., London W.C.I., 1970, 87.

United Nation's Report, 1987.

Virgina, H. *Basic Principles of Nursing Care.* International Council of Nurses, London, 1961, 3.

Viteless, M.S. *Industrial Psychology.* Norton, New York, 1932, 27.

Vroom, V.H. *Work and Motivation.* Wiley Eastern Ltd., New York, 1964.

Water Act, 1984.

Women in Employment (1901–56) : A joint study by the London Bureau, Simla and Employment Division, Planning Commission, 1958.

World Health Organisation, 1988.

Wyatt, S., Frassu, J.A. and Stock F.G.L. *The effects of monotony in work.* Industrial Fatigue Research Board Report (56), London, H.M. Stationary Office, 1929, 42.

Index

P

Q

R

S